A PATIENT'S GUIDE TO ACUPUNCTURE

A Patient's Guide to
ACUPUNCTURE

Everything You Need to Know

Sarah Swanberg, MS LAc

ALTHEA
PRESS

This book is intended to provide an overview of acupuncture treatment and answer any questions you might have about the theories and methods behind this ancient healing practice. This book is not intended as an educational textbook or reference tool for practitioners or as a guide for self-diagnosis or practice, and it should not be used as such.

Acupuncture may not be right for everyone, especially those with a history of fainting or seizures, with bleeding disorders or metal allergies or with pacemakers. Please consult a licensed practitioner to discuss if acupuncture is right for you.

Interior and Cover Designer: Michael Cook
Art Manager: Sue Smith
Editor: Rachel Feldman
Production Editor: Erum Khan

Illustration: © Milagri/Shutterstock, cover and pp. ii, vi, x, 1-2, 18, 42, 56-58; © 2019 Joe McKendry, pp. 13, 48, 51, 64, 67, 69, 75, 78; © Nanang R.A/Shutterstock, p. 20; © ananaline/Shutterstock, p. 22; © Peter Hermes Furian/Shutterstock, p. 29; © ellepigrafica/shutterstock, p. 53; © Tyler Olson/shutterstock, p. 55.

ISBN: Print 978-1-64152-559-6 | eBook 978-1-64152-560-2

R1

For Randie, my favorite person and
my biggest supporter,
and Sadie & Remy, my proudest achievements
and my smallest teachers

Contents

Introduction

Hello! If you've picked up this book, you're probably interested in learning a bit about acupuncture and are curious if it could work for you. Or maybe you're already receiving acupuncture and want to know more about how and why it works. Perhaps you're considering studying acupuncture and want to learn the basics from a patient's perspective before taking the leap. Whatever the reason, I'm so glad you're here. I'm excited to share the wisdom of this powerful, ancient practice with you.

I fell in love with acupuncture in my twenties, but before that I knew nothing about Chinese medicine. In fact, I was pretty immersed in the conventional mainstream medical model. At age seven, I was diagnosed with type 1 diabetes, an autoimmune condition that requires daily injections of insulin and several doctors' visits a year. I now receive a constant flow of my medication through an insulin pump and use devices that monitor my blood sugar for me. Advances in technology and Western medicine have allowed me to live a full and active life, and I am so thankful for that. But when I discovered Chinese medicine, my eyes were opened to an entirely new way of understanding health. In Chinese medicine, health is not just lab values—it is a complex integration of physical, emotional, and environmental factors, and this holistic way of approaching health has helped me heal in different ways.

My first experience with acupuncture came while visiting a college friend who had left her premed program to study Chinese medicine in San Diego. I flew out to visit her and received an acupuncture treatment for some airplane-induced cranky back pain. I was impressed (and a little surprised) when, thanks to a few well-placed, painless needles, the pain completely disappeared. Later, a friend of hers, also an acupuncture student, asked to see my tongue and made some spot-on assumptions about my health. I thought it was fascinating, and it showed me how Chinese medicine can fill some of the gaps in Western medicine. Years later, I began receiving regular acupuncture to help with sleep and anxiety, and I was intrigued when I realized that, along with these issues, my digestion, PMS, and energy began to improve.

My fascination and desire to learn more is what led me to enroll in a four-year program at Pacific College of Oriental Medicine in New York City. The program, a Master of Science in Traditional Oriental Medicine, covered all the tenets of Chinese medicine—acupuncture, herbology, cupping, and moxibustion—while also providing a comprehensive overview of biomedicine, including anatomy, physiology, and pharmacology. Since then I've graduated, passed all of the national board exams, had two daughters, continued my studies in both Chinese and Western medicine, and built my dream practice in Stamford, Connecticut. In my clinic, I treat pain, infertility, anxiety, and everything in between.

This book is intended to help answer many of the questions you might have. It covers the basics of acupuncture and diagnosis from a Chinese medicine perspective in a way that's comprehensive but also easy to understand. I'll go over the history, the fundamental theories, and some of the terms you might hear when in an acupuncturist's office. I'll guide you on how to find a qualified acupuncturist and provide clarity on what you can expect during your treatment. I'll also discuss some of the ailments most commonly treated with acupuncture and provide some DIY acupressure points you can try at home.

The theories and philosophies I discuss in this book are simplified to give you the broad view of how health works in Chinese medicine; keep in mind that there are nuances and intricate concepts that can take years to learn and decades to master. This book is just the tip of the iceberg. If you're curious and want to learn more, check out the Resources section at the end of the book (page 90).

I am so lucky to be one of those people who truly loves what they do, and I am excited to be sharing this gift with you. Good luck on your journey!

Part One

A Patient's Primer
on Acupuncture

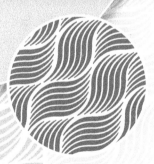

Chapter One

Introducing Acupuncture

ACUPUNCTURE, THE PRIMARY THERAPEUTIC METHOD of Chinese medicine, has been practiced for more than 2,000 years, yet it has only recently been gaining popularity in Western societies. When acupuncture first garnered interest in the United States in the early 1970s, many skeptics believed it was only a matter of time before modern scientific methods would be able to disprove the existence of acupuncture points and meridians. They were quite wrong. Acupuncture has stood the test of time, and now it is standing the test of science.

Our modern healthcare systems are in a state of crisis, and despite the principles and philosophies of Chinese medicine still not being well understood by most Western minds, interest in the effective and time-honored practice of acupuncture is growing. In fact, it's more mainstream now than it's ever been before. These days it's not uncommon to see acupuncture being discussed in *The New York Times*, being praised by celebrities like Kim Kardashian and Robert Downey Jr., and—more excitingly—being recommended by doctors and other conventional healthcare providers. So, you may be wondering, what's all the hubbub about? What does acupuncture really involve? How does it work? Does it hurt? And can it really help me?

This chapter explores all of these questions and more. There's so much to learn about acupuncture and the theories behind it—we'll only be scratching the surface in this book! But you'll learn everything you need to know about being a patient, starting with my favorite question: "So, you're really going to stick a bunch of needles in me, leave the room, and that's going to help?" (Yes, it is, and you'll probably love it.)

What Is It?

Acupuncture is one of the primary treatments under the umbrella of Chinese and East Asian medicine, and it's been around for a very long time. Its first mention in writing was around 100 BCE, but many scholars believe its use goes back several centuries before that. Despite its long history in the East, acupuncture has only been accessible in the United States for a relatively short time. While early users of acupuncture in the West touted its efficacy, it has taken a long time for popularity to heat up.

The philosophies of Chinese medicine differ greatly from what many of us grew up with in the West, and translation issues have compounded the general mistrust and confusion. This has led many Westerners to argue that acupuncture is just a placebo, meaning that you need to "believe" in it for it to work. (I like to tell skeptical friends that acupuncture is *nothing* like the tooth fairy . . . it works whether you believe in it or not.)

The treatment itself involves the insertion of hair-thin needles at specific points on the body to promote balance and healing. I'll get more into the how and why in later chapters, but here's a brief overview: In Chinese medicine, health depends on a delicate balance of Yin and Yang in the body. Yin and Yang become imbalanced when the flow of Qi (pronounced *chee)* becomes interrupted or blocked. Qi—a very important concept in acupuncture—is the life force that regulates all of the body's processes. It flows through meridians, or channels, in the body to the 12 organs, which have more to do with function than physical form (you will see these organs capitalized throughout the book to make this distinction). Any interruption or blockage in the flow of Qi in one of the 12 organs or its corresponding meridian can cause an imbalance of Yin and Yang and lead to illness. This balance of Yin and Yang relates very closely to the Western idea of homeostasis— the delicate balance of all of the body's systems, which is essential to maintaining health.

But as any acupuncturist will tell you, acupuncture involves far more than just the insertion of needles. Chinese medicine utilizes a much more holistic approach than most modern Western medicine, which tends to be more segmented and specialized. Whereas a conventional Western medicine practitioner would identify and treat a symptom, an acupuncturist will take note of the symptom, and then, like a good detective, use that as a clue to identify a pattern of imbalance in the body that may be causing your symptoms. (A "pattern" refers to a grouping of symptoms.)

As you'll see in part 2 of this book, one symptom, such as a headache, can have several possible patterns of imbalance. It's the job of the acupuncturist to seek out the root cause by asking questions, observing the tongue, and taking the pulse. We call this method of diagnosis "root and branch" identification, and it is the key to effective acupuncture treatment. The *root* is the underlying cause, while the *branch* is the presenting symptom.

The Five Most Common Questions

Does acupuncture hurt? Acupuncture needles are hair-thin filiform needles (not the hollow syringes used for injections or drawing blood), and their insertion is virtually painless. Points on the hands and feet can sometimes feel a little sharp, but the sensation is brief. It is not uncommon to feel warmth or a dull ache around the point after the needle is inserted, and you might even feel a slight pulling sensation—this is called *de Qi* ("grabbing of the Qi"), and many people enjoy the way it feels. Once the needling is finished, most people feel a sense of deep calm and relaxation, similar to a daydream state. (I call this the acu-nap!)

What are the risks? Licensed acupuncturists receive thorough training in needling technique and safety, which means that risks of serious side effects are *very* small. The most common side effects are minor bleeding and bruising at the needle site or dizziness after a treatment. More serious—but *extremely* rare—complications include organ puncture and nerve damage. Acupuncture may not be suitable for people on blood-thinner medications, with pacemakers, or with a history of fainting and seizures.

How much does it cost? Private acupuncture, the most common style of treatment, can run anywhere from $70 to $150 per session. Community acupuncture, typically performed in a shared open space in recliner chairs, is becoming a popular and cost-effective option at about $30 to $50 a session, with many of these spaces offering sliding-scale or income-based rates. Several health insurance plans now cover acupuncture, so I recommend checking with your insurer to see if you qualify for coverage.

How many sessions will I need? The number of sessions you'll need depends on your ailment and how long you've had it. In general, the more chronic the issue, the longer the course of treatment. Because your acupuncturist is working to restore balance and promote your body's own healing mechanisms, it can take time to see results. I typically recommend weekly treatments for four to six weeks before judging if acupuncture is helping.

What can it treat? Here's the general rule: If your condition can improve, acupuncture can help. The most common issues people see an acupuncturist for are anxiety, insomnia, headaches, digestive issues, fertility and hormonal issues, and pain. While acupuncture can help reduce pain and inflammation after an injury, it is always wise to have an evaluation by a medical doctor to rule out fractures and structural damage before trying acupuncture.

Who Is It For?

Acupuncture is slow but effective medicine; it helps by promoting balance in the body and by stimulating the body's own healing abilities. Conventional Western medicine, on the other hand, excels at treating acute, emergency conditions. If you've been suffering from a chronic illness and haven't found relief from conventional Western medicine, give acupuncture a try. If you're in pain and want to avoid dangerous painkillers, acupuncture could help. If you're hoping to get pregnant or want natural solutions for insomnia and anxiety, acupuncture might be your answer. And if you are feeling great and want to stay that way—check out acupuncture! You probably see where I'm going with this: There isn't much that acupuncture can't help with, and in the hands of a properly trained acupuncturist, there are very few risks, so it is always worth trying.

Always let your acupuncturist know the full extent of your medical history. They especially need to know if you have a chronic illness, are pregnant, take blood-thinner medications, have a history of fainting or seizures, or use a pacemaker, as this information may affect your treatment.

The following are some of the most common reasons people seek out acupuncture treatment. For more information on specific conditions, see chapter 4 (page 58).

Mental and Emotional Conditions: Because Chinese medicine presents a unique view of the body where emotions are closely tied to specific organs, acupuncture can be very helpful in working with mental and emotional conditions. The most common ones I see in the office are anxiety, depression, insomnia, and irritability. I work with patients both on and off medications and often receive referrals from therapists and psychiatrists who are looking for additional tools to help support their patients.

Physical Conditions: Research has shown acupuncture's effectiveness in reducing both acute and chronic pain. The insertion of a needle at an area of pain can help relax the muscle and promote blood flow to the tissue, promoting healing. Research shows that acupuncture increases the circulation of the body's natural painkillers, called endorphins. Commonly treated pain conditions include back and neck pain, frozen shoulder, knee pain, headaches, menstrual pain, and abdominal pain.

Acute Infections and Viral Conditions: As you'll learn in chapter 2, Chinese medicine looks at acute viral and bacterial infections (like the common cold and flu) as a combination of two factors: the strength of the external pathogens and the strength of a patient's protective Qi, called Wei Qi (pronounced *way chee*). Using points that help resolve illness by clearing pathogens and by supporting proper flow of Wei Qi in the body, acupuncture has long been used to both prevent and treat colds and flus. Acupuncture can help shorten the duration of a cold, open up congested nasal passages, reduce headache and throat pain, and promote recovery.

Long-Term Chronic Illnesses: While conventional Western medicine is great at treating acute, emergency conditions, it sometimes leaves patients who have chronic illnesses feeling frustrated. Chinese medicine is often able to see underlying patterns of disharmony that aren't as clear through a Western lens. Acupuncture is very helpful in treating autoimmune conditions, gastrointestinal issues like irritable bowel syndrome (IBS) and inflammatory bowel disorder (IBD), chronic fatigue syndrome, and asthma—as well as helping with the anxiety, fatigue, and stress that come with dealing with a chronic illness.

Preventive Treatment: Much like a car tune-up that checks to make sure everything is running smoothly, regular acupuncture treatments can keep Qi moving properly to help prevent illness and can catch any "under the hood" problems before they get worse. Most people seek out acupuncture for treatment of a specific concern, but once those issues have been addressed, I often recommend that they start coming in for monthly or seasonal "tune-ups" to prevent future issues.

A Brief History

The popularity of acupuncture in the United States is in its infancy, but the history of this medicine around the globe spans thousands of years. The exact origin of acupuncture is unknown, and due to the age and condition of the ancient texts, some of the time lines are vague. The first recorded mention of acupuncture was in the oldest known classical texts of Chinese medicine in approximately 100 BCE. Acupuncture was first popularized in the United States in the 1970s and has become increasingly prevalent and accepted over the past few decades. As the body of scientific evidence supporting acupuncture grows, more and more people are including it as a regular part of their healthcare routine.

Origins and Early Development

The *Huang Di Nei Jing* (*The Inner Canon of the Yellow Emperor*), often called the *Nei Jing*, is believed to have been compiled between 300 and 100 BCE and is regarded as the oldest book on Chinese medicine. It became the structural blueprint for all Chinese medicine methods and theories. *The Systematic Classic of Acupuncture and Moxibustion*, dated approximately 300 CE, was the first known book explaining acupuncture techniques and describing acupuncture point locations. The export of this book to Japan and Korea is believed to be the basis of other East Asian styles of acupuncture that developed over the next several centuries. Several other texts were published after 300 CE that continued to develop and support the theories and methods of acupuncture and Chinese medicine.

As techniques and principles of acupuncture were refined over the next several hundred years, acupuncture (along with herbal medicine) became the standard method of healthcare in China. In 1601, *The Great Compendium of Acupuncture and Moxibustion* was published. This encyclopedic text, the most significant book of this time period, compiled all existing works on acupuncture. It described and illustrated meridians and point locations, as well as point functions, and it became the basis of all modern-day educational textbooks on acupuncture.

Decline and Resurgence

In the mid-1800s, European missionaries began arriving in China, bringing with them new ideas about science and the body. These missionaries introduced new medical interventions, ideas about sanitation, and surgical techniques that had, until then, been completely unknown in China. The introduction of these concepts made a huge impact on public health, and they slowly began to eclipse the popularity of Chinese medicine. In 1929, in an effort to continue modernization and gain international status, China's national committee on public health voted to completely abolish Chinese medicine.

While never completely abandoned, acupuncture remained unpopular (and somewhat taboo) until 1949, when the Communist Party took over under the leadership of Mao Zedong, who hoped to unite China behind its traditional values. Over the next decade, he advocated for the use of both Western and Chinese medicine.

By this point, most medical professionals had been drawn out of smaller towns and outlying provinces to work in Western hospitals in the major cities, leaving rural areas with virtually no healthcare. Mao recognized that the economic prosperity of the country rested on the health of the agricultural workers in these areas, so in the early 1960s, he created a plan to send physicians out into the country to train farmers and peasants in a combination of both acupuncture and paramedical techniques for emergencies and basic healthcare. Those who were trained became known as "barefoot doctors." The mobilization of the barefoot doctors contributed to a steep decrease in infant mortality and raised overall life expectancy throughout the provinces. The use of acupuncture and Chinese medicine became popular in China once again.

In a continued effort to stay modern and relevant, Mao advocated for the removal of the more esoteric and spiritual aspects of the medicine, transforming it into what we call Traditional Chinese Medicine (TCM) today. Some acupuncturists still practice according to the more esoteric version of Chinese medicine, called Classical Chinese Medicine. The methods and practices discussed in this book focus on the more modernized techniques of TCM.

International Interest

In the nineteenth century, acupuncture had already slowly begun making its way west to Europe, but it wasn't until the late twentieth century that acupuncture became well known in the United States. The rise in popularity of acupuncture in America is largely credited to a *New York Times* article written in July 1971 by reporter James Reston. This article chronicled Reston's emergency appendectomy and subsequent acupuncture treatments at a Chinese hospital in Beijing, where he was covering a visit by Secretary of State Henry Kissinger. His observations on the effectiveness of acupuncture for his postsurgical pain generated curiosity in the United States, and interest began to grow. In 1975 the New England School of Acupuncture, the first of its kind, opened in Boston, Massachusetts, and several other teaching universities opened in the following years.

In 1991, the U.S. Congress voted to establish the Office of Alternative Medicine, known today as the National Center for Complementary and Integrative Health, further validating the use of acupuncture, and in 1997, the National Institutes of Health (NIH) released a consensus report on the use and effectiveness of acupuncture for a variety of conditions. This report concluded that, despite issues with research quantity and quality, acupuncture may be useful as an adjunct treatment or an acceptable alternative treatment for several conditions, including postoperative pain, osteoarthritis, headaches, and menstrual pain. In 2003, the World Health Organization (WHO) released a list of conditions that it found, based on a review of literature, to be effectively treated by acupuncture. In 2017, the Acupuncture Evidence Project expanded this list to include 117 conditions.

Treatment Today

In the last two decades, acupuncture has evolved from a fringe treatment to an integral (but sometimes controversial) part of modern healthcare. Today, acupuncture is covered by numerous health insurance plans, and many hospitals employ acupuncturists in integrative healthcare settings for everything from oncology to pain management.

The U.S. military trains medics in "battlefield" acupuncture, and through the Veterans Choice and Accountability Act of 2014, military veterans are able to obtain acupuncture services free of charge. With the threat of the opioid epidemic growing quickly, many medical doctors refer their patients for acupuncture treatment before prescribing potentially dangerous painkillers. Major hospitals, including Boston Children's Hospital, Kaiser Permanente, and the Mayo Clinic, as well as Veterans Affairs hospitals, all list acupuncture among their services, moving acupuncture from the strictly "alternative" medicine world into an integrative model. This gives patients access to the best of both worlds.

Celebrities including Kim Kardashian, Matt Damon, Gwyneth Paltrow, and Robert Downey Jr. have expressed their appreciation for acupuncture and have helped shine a spotlight on it, bringing it into mainstream popularity. Celebrities and other influencers who have used their social media platforms to discuss their acupuncture treatments have led to a greater awareness and public demand for acupuncture.

This increased demand for acupuncture has led to a growth of the profession, both in the number of people graduating from acupuncture programs every year and in the number of clinics available in bigger cities as well as in rural areas of the country. The continued acceptance of acupuncture and the movement toward integrative medicine in mainstream hospital care is leading acupuncture toward a bright future.

Western Research

Some Chinese medicine purists reject the notion of trying to prove that acupuncture works by Western methods. Their argument is that clinical and anecdotal evidence (that is, that it's been helping people feel better for millennia) is enough. They further argue that trying to translate Chinese medicine philosophies and define Qi in scientific terms is completely missing the point (pun intended). That being said, research helps Western minds understand and trust Chinese medicine more, which is an important step in getting acupuncture universally included in hospital care and insurance coverage.

As our ability to study the body in more detail has grown, so too has the evidence supporting acupuncture. We know that acupuncture works, but we are still learning exactly how. There are many theories about the mechanism of action behind acupuncture. Here are a few of them:

- One major hypothesis is that acupuncture works by stimulating neurohormonal pathways in the body, promoting the release and regulation of neurotransmitters, endorphins, hormones, and other important chemicals and allows the body to move out of sympathetic (fight-or-flight) mode and into parasympathetic mode, which is responsible for rest, relaxation, digestion, and healing. Using functional MRIs of the brain, scientists have found that the insertion of a needle at specific acupuncture points modulates brain activity in the limbic system and subcortical structures.
- Another hypothesis is that acupuncture helps reduce pro-inflammatory markers in the body, which decreases inflammation and pain. Scientists have been able to see that the most powerful acupuncture points on the body are located at the site of small bundles of nervous system tissue.
- In his book *The Spark in the Machine*, British physician Daniel Keown theorizes that the acupuncture meridians are actually electrical pathways found in the connective tissue in the body called fascia.

It's possible that all of these theories are correct, but there's also much more we still need to understand. Modern research into acupuncture is ongoing, but it is complicated by the fact that studying acupuncture interventions is pretty tricky. The gold standard for biomedical research is the double-blind randomized controlled trial. In a study like this, participants are randomly split into two groups. One group is given the intervention, usually a pharmaceutical medication. The other group is given a placebo, or sugar pill. Neither the participants nor the researchers know who is given the drug or the placebo until the trial is complete. This reduces any interference of psychological bias.

These studies work well for drugs, but not for acupuncture. First of all, it's impossible to perform a double-blind acupuncture study. Both the practitioner *and* the patient know if the patient is receiving acupuncture. Second, it requires all patients to receive the same treatments, which completely disregards the fundamentals of a personalized Chinese medicine diagnosis. The size, quality, and financial backing of studies all play a role, too. Despite these issues, several high-quality studies *have* shown the efficacy of acupuncture over the past few decades; the References section on page 91 has a good sampling of them, and these are the studies I refer to throughout this book.

Thanks to modern medical interventions like surgery and antibiotics, we are able to live longer, healthier lives. But many would argue that this is a sick-care system and that these therapies don't do much to *prevent* disease and can sometimes cause a cascade of other issues. Acupuncture is stepping in to fill some of the gaps in our healthcare system.

Other Treatments

While acupuncture is the most well-known modality of Chinese medicine, there are several other techniques under this umbrella, including gua sha ("scraping"), moxibustion, cupping, and acupressure. There are also more modern techniques like electroacupuncture, which uses electric currents to stimulate needles, and ear acupuncture. Your acupuncturist might use some of these techniques in conjunction with, or as an alternative to, acupuncture. The non-needle techniques mentioned below often provide a great starting point for children or for people terrified by the idea of needles.

Electroacupuncture

Electroacupuncture is the use of electric current applied directly to pairs of needles after they are inserted into the body. Studies suggest that electroacupuncture can stimulate a larger area than a single needle alone, resulting in a greater output of endorphins, our natural painkillers, making it very useful for pain. The use of electricity on motor points, the areas of a muscle or tissue near the nerve innervation (where the nerve meets the muscle), sends a quick jolt into the tissue and can help "reset" a tight band or trigger point. Electroacupuncture is often used by acupuncturists who specialize in pain and orthopedic conditions.

Ear Acupuncture

Ear acupuncture, also called auriculotherapy, was developed in France in the mid-twentieth century by French neurologist Paul Nogier. Nogier studied the correspondence between the ear and the organs, and using a variety of scientific methods, he developed a detailed map of the ear that included 43 points, each corresponding to a specific organ or area of the body. These points can be used in addition to full-body acupuncture or as its own treatment for stress, pain, and other imbalances. Most notably, ear points are frequently used in the treatment of addiction—for everything from drugs to smoking to eating disorders to gambling. The effectiveness of ear points for addiction led to the creation of the National Acupuncture Detoxification Association (NADA). NADA's ear point protocol is frequently used at drug and alcohol rehabilitation facilities to reduce cravings and support recovery.

Cosmetic Acupuncture

Cosmetic acupuncture, commonly known as facial rejuvenation acupuncture, is a rapidly growing specialty offshoot of traditional acupuncture that is gaining popularity in the United States and worldwide for its antiaging benefits. It's been touted as a natural alternative to more invasive dermatological treatments like Botox and surgery. By using very fine needles placed at specific points on the face and complementary techniques like facial cupping and gua sha, cosmetic acupuncture treatments aim to increase blood flow and stimulate collagen production, promote lymph drainage, and reduce the appearance of wrinkles by either relaxing tight muscles or activating loose muscles on the face and neck.

Celebrities such as Kim Kardashian, Madonna, and Gwyneth Paltrow have all been vocal about their use of cosmetic acupuncture as part of their skin-care routines. If this is something you'd like to try, make sure your acupuncturist has received special training in cosmetic acupuncture as there may be an increased risk of bleeding and bruising.

Cupping

Cupping is a therapy in which heated glass cups or vacuum-pumped plastic cups are applied to an area of the body, usually the back or legs, creating suction to clear stagnations and encourage the movement of the vital substances Qi and Blood. The cups are left in place for several minutes and can help relax tight muscles, stimulate healing, and reduce pain.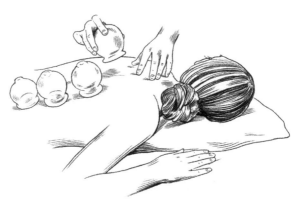
Most people describe the feeling as being similar to a "reverse" deep tissue massage. Cupping is very effective in treating chronic neck, shoulder, and back pain. It can also be helpful in the treatment of lung disorders like asthma, in which the muscles of the back often become fatigued.

Unlike bruises, which indicate a trauma to the deeper tissues in the body, cupping marks—the signature red or purple circles left behind after a cupping treatment—are normal and indicate that blood stagnation in the superficial tissue has been brought up to the surface to be cleared by the lymphatic system. The marks typically last up to a week and are not painful.

Acupressure

Acupressure is a technique in which pressure is manually applied to an acupuncture point on the body using the fingers, palms, hands, and even elbows. You can think of this as acupuncture without needles; manually stimulating these points can gently help move the vital substances Qi and Blood. While less effective than acupuncture, acupressure can still help provide relief from pain and discomfort and is often recommended for self-treatment of headaches, nausea, and motion sickness. Massage therapists and bodyworkers sometimes use acupressure during their treatments, and acupuncturists will often guide their patients in acupressure techniques to use at home. The amount of pressure to use varies depending on the location on the body, but the general rule is to apply moderate pressure on the point using small circular motions for 60 to 90 seconds.

DIY Acupressure: The Basics

You can use acupressure at home to get a better idea of how it works and to supplement your acupuncture sessions between visits. In part 2, you'll find some acupressure points to help alleviate specific issues. A great all-around point to use is *Yin Tang,* a point located right above the bridge of the nose between the eyebrows (page 64). This point helps calm the spirit. Try a bit of acupressure on this point by using the following instructions.

First, get in a comfortable seated position. Like acupuncture, acupressure also works best if you can relax and turn your mind away from any stressors. Take a few deep breaths and close your eyes. With your fingertips, apply moderate pressure to the point for 60 to 90 seconds, using circular motions. Focus on your breathing while applying pressure; deep breaths help reduce pain and stress. Allow your exhale to be slightly longer than your inhale, which helps your body relax more deeply. Use as often as needed!

Moxibustion

Moxa (dried mugwort leaves) is a commonly used Chinese herb noted for its ability to warm and move the vital substances Blood and Qi in the body; it can also be used to help stop bleeding and alleviate pain and swelling caused by Blood or Qi stagnation. Moxibustion is a Chinese medical therapy in which this herb is burned to encourage warmth and blood flow to a specific area of the body. Moxibustion can be administered with or without acupuncture. When used in conjunction with acupuncture, the moxa is often burned on or near the handle of the needle. In other cases, it may be burned on or near the skin.

Gua Sha

Similar to cupping, gua sha (pronounced *gwa sha*) is a technique used to encourage the flow of the vital substances Qi and Blood. Using a lubricating oil and a hard tool like a piece of jade or porcelain soup spoon, the practitioner will use a scraping or press-stroking technique to cause petechiae or "sha" to appear on the skin. These marks fade over time but might last up to a week. This technique helps mobilize soft tissue and reduce fascial adhesions, or scar-like tissue. In Chinese medicine, this is said to clear Qi and Blood stagnation in the tissues, and it is particularly helpful for muscle and joint pain and stiffness.

Finding a Practitioner

There are several ways to find an acupuncturist. You can find board-certified acupuncturists near you by searching the practitioner database at NCCAOM.org. Word of mouth also works really well, so ask your doctors and friends, and even do some digging on social media. In this book, I use the term *acupuncturist* to mean a licensed acupuncturist trained in Chinese medicine, but in some states, other professions can use the designation acupuncturist or can perform acupuncture. You'll want to check out the credentials of anyone who is claiming to be an acupuncturist, as discussed next.

Credentials

Acupuncture is defined as the insertion of an acupuncture needle at a specific point in the body. Not everyone who can perform acupuncture can legally call themselves an acupuncturist, and not everyone who calls themselves an acupuncturist is trained in the method of diagnosis I discuss in this book. This can create confusion for the public (not to mention a few legal issues). The degree names and license designations can vary by state. Here is what you need to know:

- Chinese medicine–trained acupuncturists receive a three- to four-year master of science or professional doctorate degree from an accredited university and are required to have more than 3,000 hours in didactic and clinical training. There are currently 57 colleges and universities in the United States accredited by the Accreditation Commission for Acupuncture and Oriental Medicine. Some schools focus less on Traditional Chinese Medicine (TCM) and more on East Asian acupuncture traditions like Japanese acupuncture or Five Element acupuncture, whereas others focus more on a modern orthopedic style of treatment. A variety of programs are available, but if your acupuncturist graduated from an accredited program in the United States, you can assume that it was a rigorous and academically thorough program.
- Almost all states require that acupuncturists take board exams to become certified with the National Certification Commission for Acupuncture and Oriental Medicine (NCCAOM) before obtaining a license. In most states, the licensed designation is Licensed Acupuncturist (LAc), but variations of this are Registered Acupuncturist (RAc, Reg. Ac.), Acupuncture Physician (AP), or Doctor of Acupuncture (DAc or D. Acu).
- Medical doctors can receive an acupuncture certification after they've taken an acupuncture training program. This is typically a 300-hour program completed over several weekends. These programs focus primarily on point location and function and do not typically include the intricate Chinese medicine pattern diagnosis discussed in this book. Medical doctors are not required to sit for acupuncture board exams or receive additional licensure. This certification is becoming popular among pain management and integrative physicians and can be helpful in treating basic ailments that might not require a full Chinese medicine pattern diagnosis.
- Some physical therapists and chiropractors can obtain a 30-hour training to perform dry needling or trigger point therapy for pain. There are valid concerns over the lack of academic standards and potential risk to public safety with such a brief training. Because of this, many states are adopting laws to ban the practice of acupuncture by anyone without a medical or acupuncture license.

Note: Some Western readers may be surprised to see the word "Oriental" still being used in proper names of medical programs, practices, etc. During the late seventies when acupuncture first became professionally recognized in the United States, the term "Oriental" was used to encompass not just acupuncture in China but also other disciplines of acupuncture practiced in Japan and Korea. Most of the schools and governing bodies that were created during that time still use the term, but many are moving away from it and beginning to replace it with "East Asian" medicine. I suspect that the term "Oriental" will die out in the near future.

Other Factors to Consider

When choosing your acupuncturist, be sure to also consider the following:

Time and Location: You will probably be seeing your acupuncturist regularly, at least in the beginning, so find someone who works near your home or workplace and has availability in their schedule that works for you.

Specialization: Keep in mind that while most acupuncturists treat all sorts of symptoms, some prefer to specialize in conditions like fertility, pregnancy, orthopedics/pain, and oncology. Before you schedule an appointment, make sure the acupuncturist you choose will be comfortable treating your condition.

Comfort: You'll be working closely with your acupuncturist and discussing emotions and everything from bowel movements to anxiety, so it's really important to work with someone you'll be comfortable sharing these details with.

Cost: Find out if you have acupuncture coverage on your insurance plan, and if you do, find an acupuncturist who accepts your plan or will provide you with a receipt that can be submitted to your insurance company for reimbursement. If your plan doesn't have coverage but you have a Health Savings Account (HSA) or Flexible Spending Account (FSA), this can often be used for acupuncture, too! If you won't be using insurance, find out how much each session will cost ahead of time. Depending on where you live, private acupuncture sessions can cost anywhere from $70 to $150 per session. For more affordable options, see if there are any community acupuncture clinics in your area that offer income-based or sliding-scale rates. Keep in mind that you'll receive acupuncture in a group setting, so you'll have to be comfortable with a lack of privacy.

Chapter Two

Principles of Acupuncture

TO UNDERSTAND HOW ACUPUNCTURE RESTORES balance and homeostasis in your body, you'll need a little working knowledge of the foundational principles of Chinese medicine discussed in this chapter. The delicate balance of these substances and concepts are the building blocks of health.

While it may be tempting to try to compare some of these principles to what we know about anatomy and physiology from a Western perspective, it's important to remember that this is a *completely* different way of thinking about the body, and many of these concepts cannot simply be translated into familiar terms. If conventional Western medicine thinks of the body as a machine, where a broken part must be fixed or replaced, Chinese medicine thinks of the body as a natural ecosystem that is dependent on many factors.

Think of it this way: For a garden to flourish, the soil properties, seed quality, sunlight, and rainwater all play an important role. External factors like frosts and parasites can negatively impact an otherwise healthy garden. If the leaves of a prized plant began to turn brown, the gardener would not simply cut off those leaves and move on—they would investigate the cause of the browning leaves and treat the root issue (and, yes, probably trim the leaves back, too). This is the way we look at the body in Chinese medicine. Identifying a symptom is not enough for treatment—the body must be viewed as a whole, and other signs and symptoms must be collected to identify a root imbalance and create an appropriate treatment plan.

You'll notice throughout this chapter that names of body parts are capitalized in Traditional Chinese Medicine to further differentiate them from their Western counterparts.

Yin and Yang

In Chinese medicine, health relies on a delicate interplay of Yin and Yang. (By the way, *Yang* rhymes with "pong"; this term is often mispronounced in the West.) Yin and Yang are used to define and explain the dynamic relationships of all things in the universe, including the human body, and they represent opposite, but complementary, parts that both depend on and balance one another.

Yin and Yang each have specific, opposing characteristics. Yin, for example, is dark, while Yang is light. Everything in the universe can be continuously divided into Yin and Yang parts. Darkness of night, while fundamentally Yin, also has Yang elements, like the moon and stars. The back of the body, while fundamentally Yang, can be divided into Yin (lower) and Yang (upper) parts.

The four vital aspects of Yin and Yang are:

1. Yin and Yang are opposites.
2. Yin and Yang depend on each other; one cannot exist without the other.
3. Yin and Yang counterbalance each other. When Yin is strong, Yang will be weak. When Yin is weak, Yang will be strong.
4. Yin and Yang exist in a constant state of flux and have the ability to transform into each other.

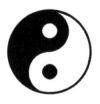

The Yin-Yang symbol provides a visual representation of these principles. Yin (black) and Yang (white) both make up half of the circle, but the S-shaped division between them represents their dynamic nature and the ability of each to transform into the other. The small white (Yang) circle inside of the Yin half represents the idea that the seed of Yang is always within Yin (and vice versa).

Yin and Yang in Acupuncture

The medical application of Yin and Yang has many facets: Areas of the body are either predominantly Yin or Yang, organs are categorized as either Yin or Yang, and illnesses have either a Yin or Yang nature. The organs that create and store substances are labeled Yin—they tend to be more solid—while the hollow organs in charge of transportation are labeled Yang. Acute illnesses are more Yang, and chronic ones are more Yin. The head is mostly Yang, whereas the lower body is mostly Yin. Because the upper body and head is Yang, these areas tend to be more easily affected by Yang factors like Wind and Heat, whereas the lower part of the torso is more Yin and thus more easily affected by Yin factors like Cold and Dampness. Everything in the universe can be broken down into Yin and Yang pairs. Here are some examples you might commonly see:

Yin	Yang
Black	White
Cold	Hot
Dark	Light
Damp	Dry
Rest	Activity
Female	Male
Lower Body	Upper Body
Front Body	Back Body
Internal	External
Winter	Summer

Optimal health in the body relies on the balance of Yin and Yang. Your acupuncturist will determine whether the imbalance you are experiencing is due to an excess or deficiency of Yin or Yang. Because Yin and Yang are so intertwined, the same symptom can stem from an excess of Yang or a deficiency of Yin, or vice versa. For example, Heat in the body can be due to an excess of Yang *or* a deficiency of Yin. In both situations, the body will display signs of Heat, but there will be a subtle distinction. If the Heat is more intense and accompanies other signs of excess like a throbbing headache, then it is *true* Heat and indicates an excess of Yang.

We see this in a case of high fever. In this case, the treatment would be to reduce Yang to clear the Heat. If the Heat is milder or intermittent and accompanies other signs of deficiency like Dryness, it is more likely to be *false* Heat, due to a deficiency of cooling Yin. This is commonly seen as night sweats and brief hot flashes during menopause. In this case, the treatment would be to nourish the Yin to clear the Heat. The following graphic illustrates the concept of true Heat and false Heat. Understanding these broad relationships and applying them to other patterns and principles can help your acupuncturist arrive at a diagnosis and treatment plan.

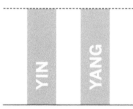

A. Balance of Yin and Yang

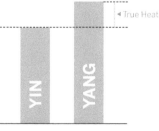

B. Excess of Yang, causing TRUE Heat

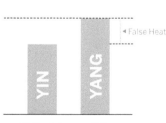

C. Deficiency of Yin, causing FALSE Heat

The Five Elements

Like Yin and Yang, the Five Element theory is used to categorize all natural phenomena into certain groupings. In this case, phenomena are categorized according to the related functions and qualities of Five Elements: Wood, Fire, Earth, Metal, and Water. Each of these elements has a set of corresponding textures, seasons, organs, times of day, stages of development, emotions, and climates.

The Five Elements interact with each other in a number of ways. As with Yin and Yang, there is a system of checks and balances among the Five Elements that ensures they exist in harmony with one another. For example, in both Five Element theory and in nature, Wood generates Fire, but it controls Earth (the roots of a tree are able to separate the ground). Water generates Wood (trees can't grow without water), but it controls (or extinguishes) Fire. The visual of the Five Element Cycle shows how intertwined the relationships among the elements are.

Important characteristics of each of the Five Elements include:

Wood is the element of growth and corresponds to the Liver and Gallbladder, the emotion anger, and the color green.

Fire is the element of maximum potential and relates to the Heart and Small Intestine, the emotion joy, and the color red.

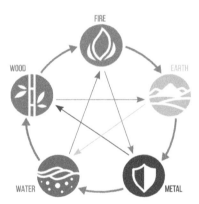

Earth is the element of stability and relates to the Spleen and Stomach, the emotion pensiveness, and the color yellow.

Metal is the element of decline and separation and relates to the Lungs and Large Intestine, the emotion sadness, and the color white.

Water is the element of stillness and relates to the Kidneys and Urinary Bladder, the emotion fear, and the colors blue and black.

The following chart can help familiarize you with the associated properties or characteristics of each of the Five Elements. Keep in mind that, as a patient, you don't need to commit this to memory.

	WOOD	FIRE	EARTH	METAL	WATER
Season	Spring	Summer	Late Summer	Autumn	Winter
Taste	Sour	Bitter	Sweet	Pungent	Salty
Climate	Wind	Heat	Dampness	Dryness	Cold
Emotion	Anger	Joy	Pensiveness	Sadness	Fear
Yin Organ	Liver	Heart	Spleen	Lungs	Kidneys
Yang Organ	Gallbladder	Small Intestine	Stomach	Large Intestine	Urinary Bladder
Sense Organ	Eyes	Tongue	Mouth	Nose	Ears
Color	Green	Red	Yellow	White	Black
Tissues	Sinews	Blood Vessels	Muscles	Skin	Bones

The Five Elements in Acupuncture

These categories can help an acupuncturist classify signs and symptoms, identify personality and constitutional types, and make connections between nature, the body, and the emotions. Some acupuncturists rely heavily on the Five Elements for diagnosis and treatment (these practitioners typically identify themselves as 5E practitioners), but other acupuncturists rely on the model solely as an organizational method to assist in grouping symptoms.

Clinically, the Five Element model can be useful in identifying patterns of disharmony. If your Wood element is deficient, your acupuncturist might use points from the meridians corresponding to Wood's generating element, Water. A common clinical example of this is an acupuncturist using Kidney (Water) meridian points to help support Liver (Wood), the organ in charge of Blood, in someone with symptoms of a Blood deficiency.

Here are a few examples of imbalance according to the Five Elements:

Wood: a green undertone in the skin, prone to outbursts of anger

Fire: blood pressure issues, heat sensitivities, and prone to inappropriate bursts of laughter

Earth: fatigue, cravings for sweets, and digestive issues

Metal: frequent respiratory illnesses, pale complexion, and tendency toward sadness

Water: fear and worry, urinary incontinence, and hearing issues

The Vital Substances

The vital substances—Qi, Essence, Blood, Body Fluids, and Shen—are the building blocks of all physiological activity in the human body. The quantity, quality, location, and balance of each substance all play a role in the balance of your health. They range from the more material substances Blood and Body Fluids, to the less material but equally important substances like Qi, Essence, and Shen. All changes that occur in the human body result from the interaction of these substances, but they are meaningful only in their relationship to other patterns and symptoms happening in your body.

Qi is the most important of all the substances, and you will hear it frequently mentioned in an acupuncturist's office. It is the force and energy of life and plays a role in all of the processes of the body. Qi is Yang in nature, propelling all movements and functions. Blood and Body Fluids are the nourishment of the body and more Yin in nature. Essence is what makes up our constitution and robustness, and it controls our growth and development. The following graphic illustrates where these four vital substances fall within the Yin-Yang continuum.

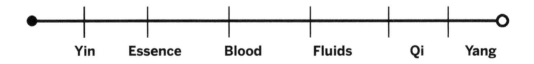

Yin Essence Blood Fluids Qi Yang

Yin-Yang Continuum of Essence, Blood, Body Fluids, and Qi. Yin substances are heavier and deeper in the body; Yang substances are lighter and circulate more rapidly.

Shen, the fifth vital substance, is our spirit, and it is what distinguishes human life from all others. Together, Shen, Essence, and Qi are known as "the three treasures"—the combination of these substances is what sustains human life.

Qi

Qi (pronounced *chee*) is by far the most important concept in Chinese medicine. The primary goal of acupuncture is to move and balance Qi in the body to restore balance and promote health. Explaining Qi succinctly is quite difficult—there is no perfect parallel for it in the English language. Qi is *everything*, and *everything* is Qi. Several of the classical texts of Chinese medicine echo the principle "When Qi gathers, the physical body is formed; when it disperses, the body dies." Qi is often translated as "vital energy" or "life force," but that only scratches the surface of what Qi is and does.

I like to think of Qi as the thread that connects the fabric of human life. It is both form and function; it is refined energy and also functional activity. It is the basis of all phenomena and can condense into physical form, while also remaining on a metaphysical level. Our bodies, for example, *are* Qi, but our bodies cannot also move *without* Qi. Qi is in a constant state of growth and decline and can be easily influenced by sleep, diet, exercise, and of course . . . acupuncture!

WHAT IT DOES

Qi in the body has many forms and functions; it circulates through the body in a series of meridians, or channels, each assigned to a master organ. (You'll learn more about the organs and meridians later in this chapter.) There are three main sources of Qi in the human body:

Source Qi: Given to us by our parents

Air Qi: Created from the air we breathe

Food Qi: Created from the food we eat

The combination of Source Qi, Air Qi, and Food Qi is called True Qi, and this is the Qi that circulates in the body. True Qi has five functions in the body:

- It is the source of all movement and activation.
- It protects against external pathogens (the role of Wei Qi).
- It controls the creation and conversion of all of the substances in the body.
- It maintains structure and keeps everything in its proper place.
- It warms the body.

Deficiency: When there is not enough Qi for proper functioning, typically due to overwork, prolonged illness, or insufficient nutrition, you may experience fatigue, shortness of breath, or frequent illness.

Sinking: Severe Qi deficiency results in sinking Qi, leading to organ prolapse (that is, the tissues or muscles supporting an organ become loose or weak).

Stagnation: When Qi stops moving properly and stagnates, it can result in pain, distention, or emotional irritability.

Rebellion: Qi flows in the wrong direction, causing symptoms like wheezing, nausea, heartburn, and headaches. Qi moving in the wrong direction is called counterflow Qi.

Essence

Essence, also known as Jing, is a substance that determines our constitution and our potential. It is primarily given to us by our parents in the form of prenatal Essence, but it also exists in combination with postnatal Essence, which is derived from food and air.

Essence is more Yin in nature than Qi and Blood, and thus it is much more difficult to affect than the other substances. The amount of Essence we receive from our parents is believed to be a fixed amount, and Essence received from our diet contributes a very small amount. There is a lot we can do to prevent the excess of Essence, but once it becomes depleted, it can be very difficult to replenish.

WHAT IT DOES

The role of Essence in the body is to promote growth, reproduction, and development, and to govern the aging process.

SIGNS OF IMBALANCE

- Delayed growth in children
- Premature aging and graying of hair
- Fragile teeth and bones
- Delayed sexual maturation or impotence
- Infertility

Blood

Despite sharing a name, Blood in Chinese medicine differs slightly from its bio-medical counterpart. Blood's characteristics are not as physically identifiable as the hemoglobin-transporting liquid that we call blood in conventional Western medicine. Blood, like Qi and Essence, is also derived in part from the food we eat. Blood is closely related to Qi and can be thought of as a denser, liquid form of it, though it still relies on Qi for movement. It is said in the classical text the *Nei Jing* that "Blood is the mother of Qi, and Qi is the commander of Blood."

WHAT IT DOES

The main roles of Blood are to nourish organs, help prevent dryness in body tissues, and allow muscles and sinews (tendons, ligaments, and cartilage) to remain supple and flexible. In addition, Blood is what anchors the Shen (see page 28) and holds it in place. The Shen can only rest when there is adequate Blood, so when Blood is deficient, the Shen floats, and symptoms like anxiety, insomnia, or dream-disturbed sleep arise.

SIGNS OF IMBALANCE

Deficiency: Blood becomes deficient due to excessive menstrual bleeding or insufficient diet. Deficient Blood can result in unsettled mental states. It can also result in pale and dry skin, dry eyes, fragile nails, stiff muscles, and menstrual irregularities.

Stagnation: Without sufficient Qi to move it, Blood can easily become stagnant. When this happens, it can result in sharp pain or heavy, crampy menstruation. Blood can also become stagnant due to an injury or trauma.

Heat: Blood can combine with Heat in the body and cause skin conditions such as acne and rashes and nosebleeds, bleeding gums, or excessive menstrual bleeding.

Body Fluids

The Chinese medicine concept of Body Fluids encompasses all the other liquids produced in the body, such as sweat, saliva, tears, urine, gastric juices, and mucus. Body Fluids originate from food and water and go through a series of intricate processes throughout different organs that separate the fluids into "pure" and "impure" forms. Pure fluids travel upward in the body and moisten the Lungs and mucous membranes and form into tears and saliva. Impure fluids travel down and are excreted as urine.

Body Fluids moisten skin, hair, and sense organs; lubricate joints; and moisten the brain. Body Fluids play a similar role to Blood in the body, and the two substances support each other. Blood is more nourishing, whereas Body Fluids are more moistening. They can easily impact each other—for example, excessive sweating can injure the Blood and heavy bleeding can cause dryness in body tissues.

SIGNS OF IMBALANCE

Deficiency: Fluid deficiency, caused by excessive sweating or insufficient hydration, results in dryness, stiffness of muscles and joints, and thirst.

Excess: Often due to an issue in the purification process, excess fluids become stagnant and cause issues like edema, swelling, excess phlegm, and mucus.

Shen

The final vital substance is the Shen. This is the fundamental texture of human life and the thing that separates us from all other creatures. It is sometimes translated to "soul" or "spirit." It is the quality in humans that allows for relationships, self-awareness, morality, and values. The Shen is visible in the eyes; when healthy, it creates a vibrant sparkle.

WHAT IT DOES

The Shen is divided into five components, each with a complex role, as follows:

Yi is consciousness, thought, and intention. It's what gives us the ability to consider and deliberate. It is the part of the spirit that allows for loyalty and faithfulness.

Hun is similar to reputation. It encompasses the good deeds of our lives and the acts of kindness that may continue to have an effect even after our death. It is benevolence and empathy, and it plays a role in our ability to endure suffering and pain.

Zhi is our willpower and intentions, and the innate wisdom we hold.

Po is our "animal" soul, the part that dies with us. This can be thought of as our instinctual and transitory emotions.

Shen-mind is the part of the Shen that allows us to properly connect with the world. It is in charge of communication and appropriateness. The Shen-mind is our consciousness, cognition, and insight. It is in charge of our sleep, ideas, memory, and worries. It also rules the five senses.

- Anxiety
- Depression
- Brain fog
- Insomnia
- When severe, mental illnesses like mania and schizophrenia

Issues of mental health will always affect the Shen, but be aware that in Traditional Chinese Medicine, mental and physical health are considered to be much more closely related than they are in conventional Western medicine (although that does seem to be changing). In Chinese medicine, each emotion is associated with a specific organ or organs. Imbalance in the emotions can be both the cause and the effect of a physical imbalance.

The Organs and the Meridians

Traditional Chinese Medicine identifies 12 major organs and corresponding meridians that work together and in combination with the vital substances to achieve balance in the body. They are illustrated here.

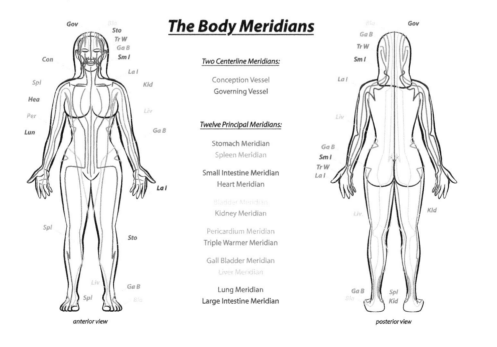

The Body Meridians

Two Centerline Meridians:

Conception Vessel
Governing Vessel

Twelve Principal Meridians:

Stomach Meridian
Spleen Meridian

Small Intestine Meridian
Heart Meridian

Bladder Meridian
Kidney Meridian

Pericardium Meridian
Triple Warmer Meridian

Gall Bladder Meridian
Liver Meridian

Lung Meridian
Large Intestine Meridian

anterior view

posterior view

Major Organs

The 12 major organs are very important to acupuncture diagnosis and treatment. In Traditional Chinese Medicine, the function of the organs is more important than their physical form, so sometimes they're very different from the organs you might normally think of. Because of this, you'll also see organs that aren't acknowledged in conventional Western medicine, like the Triple Burner (page 37).

Another big difference you'll notice is that organ names are capitalized in Traditional Chinese Medicine in an attempt to differentiate them from their Western equivalents. To make these terms more understandable to Westerners, early translators of Chinese medical texts adopted the names of the Western anatomical organs that they felt were most closely related. Unfortunately, this has contributed more to confusion than anything else (and occasionally causes an acupuncture newbie to panic and run to their primary care doctor demanding liver or heart tests). Remember: An imbalance of an organ in Chinese medicine does *not* mean that you have damage to the anatomical organ counterpart!

While many of the Chinese medicine organs share qualities with their namesake organs, some have almost no similarities. The Spleen, for example, has almost nothing in common with the biomedical spleen, and many Chinese medicine scholars believe that it is actually more closely related to the pancreas, an important digestive organ.

As discussed earlier, organs are categorized as either Yin or Yang. Yin organs create and regulate the Qi, Blood, and Body Fluids, and are each associated with a dominant emotion. Each Yin organ is paired with a complementary Yang organ that receives, processes, and absorbs food and/or promotes the transformation of fluids and substances. They also help move and excrete food particles that are not used by the body. Yin and Yang organs work in pairs to ensure that Qi and Blood circulate through the entire body.

There are six Yin organs, and they are generally thought of as more important than their Yang partners. They are the Heart, Lungs, Spleen, Liver, Kidneys, and Pericardium. You can think of these guys as the superheroes, whereas their Yang partners are the sidekicks. The six Yang organs are the Gallbladder, Stomach, Small Intestine, Large Intestine, Bladder, and Triple Burner.

Meridians

The 12 main meridians, also called channels, are each named for their master organ. They circulate Qi and Blood through the body and create a network that links all the organs and substances. Disorders of an organ can affect areas of the body linked by that organ's meridian; similarly, blockages in a meridian can affect that meridian's master organ. The 12 major meridians exist on both sides of the body, and each of them contains a series of acupuncture points that are used to manipulate the Qi flowing through them. There are two additional major meridians not associated with the organs: the Du (governing) meridian, and the Ren (conception) meridian. These meridians run up and down the midline of the body.

There are 365 regular acupuncture points on the body and countless "extra" points, but in general, an acupuncturist may use only 100 or so of these points, each with a different and very specific function.

If you've ever been to New York City, you may be familiar with the complex subway system that runs both below- and aboveground. Our meridian system works a lot like this. When all the subway lines are running smoothly and efficiently, you can easily get wherever you need to go. But if a signal goes out at Grand Central Terminal, one of the main hubs, it can cause train congestion (and unhappy passengers) as far out as Queens and the Bronx. Correcting the signals at Grand Central and making sure the signals are all timed properly at the other stations along the lines can help get trains moving properly again and restore normal service. Acupuncture points work the same way: To correct an issue, an acupuncturist often uses points close to the area of imbalance but also elsewhere along the meridians to encourage proper flow.

Liver

The **Liver organ** has several important functions, including storing Blood and promoting the smooth and gentle flow of Qi through the body. Liver Blood is important for nourishing the eyes and sinews (tendons, ligaments, and cartilage) and for regulating menstruation. The smooth flow of Liver Qi helps maintain balanced emotions, restful sleep, and healthy digestion. The Liver's sensitivity makes it especially susceptible to stress, which is why disharmonies related to Liver Qi stagnation are some of the most commonly seen patterns in an acupuncturist's office.

The **Liver meridian** begins at the big toe, travels up the inner portion of the leg, circles the genitals, and enters the lower abdomen. It then travels up the side body, over the ribs, and ends in the Lung. The Liver meridian's connection to the genitals is why points on the Liver meridian are often used to treat gynecological and testicular pain.

> **Physical signs of imbalance:** genital pain, regular or painful periods, PMS, breast distention, hiccups, headaches, dizziness, blurry vision, dry eyes

> **Emotional signs of imbalance:** anger, resentment, depression, anxiety, irritability

Gallbladder

The **Gallbladder organ** stores and secretes bile, which aids in the digestive process. Bile is created by a surplus of Blood and Qi in the Liver, the Gallbladder's paired organ. The Liver and Gallbladder have a very close relationship, and disharmonies concerning one of these organs often directly affect the other. When emotional issues like anger and frustration affect the Liver, the Liver Qi can stagnate and create Heat, which can then spill over into the Gallbladder and create additional symptoms of irritability, bitter taste, and headaches. The Gallbladder rules decisiveness and courage, so emotional issues like timidity and fear can often be due to an imbalance of the Gallbladder. It can also be easily affected by greasy and fatty foods, which cause Dampness that can lead to gallstones and jaundice.

The **Gallbladder meridian** begins at the eye and zigzags over the head before traveling down the side body, through the hip, down the outside of the front of the leg, over the ankle, and ends at the tip of the fourth toe. Because of its connection to the hip, points on the Gallbladder meridian are often used to treat hip pain and sciatica.

Physical signs of imbalance: hip pain, nausea and vomiting, rib fullness and distention

Emotional signs of imbalance: anxiety, difficulty making decisions, irritability

Lungs

The **Lung organs** control respiration and have the important job of inhaling pure Air Qi, which then becomes the basis for all other Qi in the body. Because of this, the Lungs are said to "govern" Qi. The Lungs also control the free movement of Qi and Body Fluids throughout the body and control the skin and the region between the skin and muscles. Additionally, the Lungs play a role in descending Body Fluids down to the Kidneys and Urinary Bladder, and spreading fluids out to the skin and muscles, keeping the skin moist. Sadness, worry, and grief can deplete Lung Qi, explaining why tightness in the chest occurs during periods of sorrow.

The **Lung meridian** exits the Lung and travels down the inner arm and down the hand, where it terminates at the tip of the thumb.

Physical signs of imbalance: chronic respiratory infections, asthma, shortness of breath, cough, dry skin, frequent colds and flus, allergies

Emotional signs of imbalance: unresolved grief, sadness, detachment

Large Intestine

The **Large Intestine organ** continues the work of the Small Intestine by moving impure substances down for excretion while also absorbing water to assist in the proper formation and excretion of stool. When this water absorption function is impaired, the result is either loose or dry, hard stool. Because the Large Intestine has the final job of "letting go," it can also influence our emotional capacity for letting go and not dwelling on the past.

The **Large Intestine meridian** begins at the index finger and runs up the arm and neck and ends at the nose. Points on this meridian can be used to treat thumb pain, tennis elbow, shoulder pain, headaches, and sinus congestion.

Physical signs of imbalance: constipation, diarrhea, headaches, toothaches, sinus pressure

Emotional signs of imbalance: inability to let go of the past

Spleen

The **Spleen organ** directs all upward movement and plays an important role in the creation of Qi and Blood. It is a primary organ of digestion along with its Yang partner, the Stomach, and its main job is to extract nutrition from food and fluids and aid in their transformation into Qi and Blood. If the Spleen is imbalanced, the result is often digestive symptoms such as abdominal distention, diarrhea, and low appetite combined with Qi and Blood deficiency signs like fatigue and weakness. The Spleen houses the intellect and is also responsible for thinking, pondering, and making decisions. An imbalanced Spleen may result in frequent worrying, difficulty making decisions, and mental confusion.

An additional role of the Spleen is "governing" the Blood, which allows Blood to stay in its proper path. Any bleeding not related to trauma (blood in the stool, easy bruising, excess uterine bleeding, bloody noses, etc.) is generally thought to be related to a Spleen Qi deficiency. Because of its role in the creation of Qi and Blood, the Spleen also has a relationship with the "flesh" (muscles), and proper muscle tone and flexibility fall under the command of the Spleen.

The **Spleen meridian** begins at the big toe, runs up the foot and inner leg, and through the abdominal cavity and chest, where it crosses through the throat and ends at the tongue.

Physical signs of imbalance: fatigue, inability to lose weight, low muscle tone, poor appetite, digestive disorders (especially loose stools with undigested food), abdominal distention, frequent bleeding and bruising, organ prolapse

Emotional signs of imbalance: frequent worrying, excessive thinking, mental confusion, difficulty making decisions

Stomach

The **Stomach organ** is the most important of all the Yang organs. Along with its Yin organ pair, the Spleen, the Stomach plays a central role in the creation of Qi. The Stomach receives food and drink and helps transform them into Qi. Because of this, impairments of the Stomach can have far-reaching implications. Fatigue due to Stomach and Spleen Qi deficiency is one of the most commonly seen patterns in an acupuncturist's office.

Diet is one of the main causes of disease patterns involving the Stomach, and acupuncturists will often include dietary recommendations in their treatments of Stomach-related issues. Excessive consumption of hot and spicy foods can create Stomach Heat, which manifests in intense thirst, excessive appetite, foul breath, bleeding gums, and mental restlessness or confusion. Excessive consumption of cold and raw foods and iced drinks can cause Cold invasion of the Stomach, which results in abdominal pain, cold limbs, and nausea.

Worry and excessive thinking, which both can affect the Spleen, can also damage the Stomach by causing Stomach Qi stagnation, leading to belching and nausea.

The **Stomach meridian** emerges under the eye, travels down past the nose, curves around the lips, and travels along the jawbone. It then travels up the side of the face to the corner of the forehead. A second branch exits from the jaw where it travels down the front of the neck, chest, and abdomen to the groin. The meridian continues down the outer leg and ends at the foot. The Stomach meridian's relationship to the face makes it helpful for treating headaches, jaw pain, and mouth issues.

Physical signs of imbalance: abdominal pain, bloating, diarrhea, constipation, vomiting, fatigue, weak limbs, low or excessive appetite

Emotional signs of imbalance: mania, confusion

Heart

The **Heart organ** is considered the most vital of all the internal organs and is often called the "emperor" of all the organs. The Heart's major function is to supply Blood to all body tissues and to control the blood vessels. The Qi of the Heart is reflected in the state of the blood vessels. If the Heart Qi is strong, the pulse will be strong and regular. If it is weak, the pulse may be weak and irregular. The Heart manifests in the complexion of the face, and strong Heart Qi will be visible in a rosy and healthy complexion.

The Heart is the organ that houses the Shen. All mental activity and consciousness are directly tied to the Heart, and the Heart plays an important role in memory, sleep, and thought. The Heart relates to the emotion of joy and also plays a role in controlling proper sweating.

The **Heart meridian** extends from the anatomical heart, exits the armpit, runs down the inner side of the arm, and ends at the pinky finger.

Physical signs of imbalance: palpitations, insomnia, unusual sweating, poor memory

Emotional signs of imbalance: depression, anxiety, inappropriate laughter, mental restlessness

Small Intestine

The **Small Intestine organ** pairs with the Heart and has the job of separating the "pure" from the "impure" fluids, continuing the job of the Stomach. The pure fluids are sent to the Spleen to be used in the creation of Qi and Blood, while the impure fluids continue downward to the Large Intestine, Kidney, and Bladder for excretion. Disharmonies of the Small Intestine may cause abdominal pain, diarrhea, and constipation. Because of its role in separation, the Small Intestine controls discernment, judgment, and clarity of thought.

The **Small Intestine meridian** begins on the outside of the pinky finger, travels up the hand, over the wrist, and up the back of the arm. It zigzags over the shoulder before crossing to the front of the body, where it extends up the neck and onto the face, ending at the ear. Because of its relationship with the shoulder, the Small Intestine meridian is used to effectively treat shoulder pain.

Physical signs of imbalance: abdominal pain, shoulder pain, diarrhea, constipation

Emotional signs of imbalance: difficulty making decisions and poor mental clarity

Kidneys

The **Kidney organs** are in command of storing Essence and rule birth, growth, and development. They are considered the root of Yin and Yang energies of the body. The role of storing Essence means that the Kidneys play an important role in constitution, vitality, sexual maturation, and fertility and influence the brain, teeth, and bones. The Kidneys have a Five Element relationship to water; issues of fluid regulation like edema and frequent urination are tied to Kidney imbalances. The Kidneys house willpower and are easily affected by fear.

The **Kidney meridian** begins under the foot, runs up the inside of the leg to the groin, and travels up the torso, ending under the collarbone. Because the kidneys are found in the lower back, low back pain is often attributed to a Kidney Qi or Yang deficiency.

Physical signs of imbalance: infertility, delayed puberty, delayed growth, premature graying of hair, fragile bones and teeth, night sweats, frequent urination, low back and knee pain

Emotional signs of imbalance: fear, low willpower, isolation, insecurity

Urinary Bladder

The **Urinary Bladder organ** is partnered with the Kidneys, and its sole function is to receive and excrete urine.

The **Urinary Bladder meridian** is the longest meridian of the body. It starts at the eye, travels over the top of the head, and has two paths down the back and upper leg. Once reaching the knee, the Urinary Bladder meridian travels down the center of the calf muscle and then moves to the outside of the leg toward the ankle, ending at the outer tip of the little toe. Because of its relationship to the back, the Urinary Bladder meridian is often used for treating back pain. Due to this organ's role of "holding on" to urine, imbalances here can lead to an emotional "holding on," linking it to grudges and jealousy.

Physical signs of imbalance: back pain, bladder pain, urinary incontinence

Emotional signs of imbalance: fear, jealousy, holding on to grudges

Pericardium

The form and function of the **Pericardium organ** is less clearly defined than other Yin organs but has a very close relationship to the Heart and acts as an outer covering/protector of the Heart. Its main function is to protect the Heart. Its other roles are similar to those of the Heart—it helps govern Blood and house the Shen. The Pericardium has a strong influence on our mental-emotional state and is responsible for relationships and connections with others.

The **Pericardium meridian** starts in the chest, travels down the inner arm and through the palm, and ends at the tip of the middle finger. Points on the Pericardium meridian can help move and cool Blood as well as influence the mind and are often used in combination with Heart meridian points.

Physical signs of imbalance: chest pain

Emotional signs of imbalance: depression, social anxiety, agitation

Triple Burner

The **Triple Burner organ** is also known as the Triple Warmer, or by its Chinese name, San Jiao. There is a lot of controversy about this organ, but it is generally agreed that the Triple Burner has "a name but no shape." Its job is to control the transportation of Qi and regulate the waterways of the body. While some Chinese medicine scholars do consider this its own organ, others consider it more of a pathway that connects different areas of the body and allows for Qi movement and waterway regulation.

The three burners—upper, middle, and lower—each have distinct roles in water movement. The upper burner is a "mist" and supports the function of the Lungs in moisturizing the skin and other organs. The middle burner is a "foam," which refers to the digestive juices and churning of the Stomach and Spleen. The lower burner is a "swamp," and its main role is the excretion of "impure" substances.

The Triple Burner also demarcates three regions of the body: The upper refers to the head and chest, the middle refers to the area between the chest and the navel, and the lower refers to everything below the navel.

The **Triple Burner meridian** begins at the back of the hand, runs up the back of the arm, then over the shoulder and up the neck to the back of the ear, before terminating at the eyebrow. Because it runs through the ear, points on the Triple Burner meridian can help treat ear pain.

Because the Triple Burner has no form, it has no imbalances or diseases directly associated with it, but it is often implicated in issues with the transformation of Body Fluids.

The Seven Emotions

As mentioned, Chinese medicine places a great emphasis on emotional balance in the body. While conventional Western medicine understands that there's a connection between mind and body, Chinese medicine considers them to be one, with no separation at all. Each emotion is thought to be stored in an organ of the body. An imbalance of emotions can negatively impact health, and health can negatively impact emotions.

The seven emotions identified in Chinese medicine are anger, joy, fear, fright (more extreme than fear), sadness, worry, pensiveness, and shock. These emotions are all considered normal and necessary but can cause disease when they either last too long or are too intense. You might be wondering how it might be a problem for joy to be too intense or last too long, as joy is generally regarded as a wonderful emotion. When joy becomes pathological, behaviors like mania and uncontrollable/inappropriate laughter occur.

These are the seven emotions and their correlated organs:

1. Anger: Liver
2. Joy: Heart
3. Fear: Kidneys
4. Fright: Kidneys/Heart
5. Sadness: Lungs
6. Worry: Spleen/Lungs
7. Pensiveness: Spleen

Each of these emotions is "stored" in its respective organ. Predominance of a particular emotion can cause imbalances in the paired organ, and vice versa. We often see issues with anger stemming from stagnation in the Liver, and unresolved grief and sadness can take a toll on the Lungs, causing a Lung Qi deficiency and resulting in asthma or chronic respiratory infections.

External Factors

Traditional Chinese Medicine differentiates all diseases as being either internal or external. Internal diseases are due to an imbalance in organs, as discussed. External diseases are caused by an imbalance between the body and the environment. There are six external factors that have the ability to impact health. They are Wind, Cold, Heat, Dryness, Dampness, and Summer Heat. A healthy body with strong protective Qi (Wei Qi) should be able to withstand normal weather changes, but if the Wei Qi is weak or if the climatic factor is excessive or inappropriate, disease can manifest.

When these climatic factors influence disease, these factors are known as external pathogens. The identification of the external pathogens was based on observation of their physical effects on the body by Chinese physicians and scholars. Wind illnesses, for example, come on quickly and move through the body with speed, whereas Dampness creates a boggy sensation in the body, leading to fatigue and bloating. (It *is* possible for some of these factors to be generated internally, as well. Dryness, for example, can also be caused by fluid loss or insufficient hydration, and Dampness can be created by a deficiency of Spleen Qi.) It's also important to note that these pathogens can combine. For example, arthritis is typically differentiated into a Wind-Damp-Cold or a Wind-Damp-Heat pattern.

Here are some common symptoms of each of the six external pathogens:

Wind: Wind presents itself as illness that comes on quickly and may include sneezing, runny nose, watery eyes, and an aversion to wind. It is usually caused by exposure to windy weather or by sleeping too close to a fan or AC unit. This is why acupuncturists always recommend wearing a scarf on windy days! Wind is usually combined with either Cold or Heat. (Wind illnesses are most closely related to what we know in conventional Western medicine as bacterial and viral infections.)

Cold: Cold presents itself as subjective or objective sensations of cold, with signs like chills, shivering, pain, cold limbs, cramps, and spasms. These signs may be caused by exposure to extreme cold or a Cold pathogen, or intake of overly cold foods, especially in the winter. Interestingly, antibiotics, which are considered Cold in nature due to their ability to fight Heat pathogens, can cause Cold in the Stomach, leading to digestive issues.

Heat: Heat presents itself as subjective or objective sensations of heat, with signs like fever, sweating, red face, red eyes, thirst, itching, and dark urine. These signs may be caused by exposure to heat or a Heat pathogen, or too much intake of spicy foods, alcohol, and sugar.

Dryness: Dryness presents itself as withering or shriveling and can be seen in the skin but also as dry cough, thirst, and constipation. This is caused by dry and/or hot environments, or because of extreme fluid or blood loss.

Dampness: Dampness typically combines with Heat or Cold and presents itself as fatigue, edema, sticky mucus, and/or cloudy urine. Dampness is usually caused by living in a damp environment or by humid weather but can also be caused by a Spleen Qi deficiency or overeating Damp-producing foods like dairy and gluten. When Dampness lingers over time, it can congeal into Phlegm, a more substantial form of Dampness.

Summer Heat: This only occurs when exposed to prolonged or extreme heat; symptoms are similar to heatstroke and include nausea, vomiting, and dizziness.

Lifestyle Factors

Lifestyle factors play a major role in disease; they could take up an entire book of their own. Most acupuncturists will include dietary and lifestyle modifications in their treatment plans to support your overall health and well-being. Here are some of the common factors your acupuncturist will consider when developing your treatment plan:

Work: Exhaustion due to being overworked is a major cause of disease, especially in the United States and other Western countries. Hectic lifestyles and long hours combined with lack of rest, poor diet, and emotional stress have taken a toll on our health. When the balance between activity and rest is off, Qi becomes depleted. Replenishing Qi requires proper nourishment but also rest to allow the Spleen and Stomach to properly convert food into Qi. If the balance between activity and rest remains unbalanced for a long time, Qi cannot be adequately restored, which can lead to disease.

Physical Activity: Excessive physical activity can similarly deplete the stores of Qi and tax the Spleen and Liver, which control the muscles and sinews (tendons, ligaments, and cartilage). Insufficient physical activity, on the other hand, can lead to a stagnation of Qi and Blood, which can also cause illness.

Sexual Activity: As mentioned earlier, we have a relatively finite amount of Essence, one of the vital substances, that determines our sexual maturation, fertility, and growth. Excessive sexual activity can deplete our stores of Essence and can lead to premature aging. I'm guessing you're wondering exactly *how much* sex is considered excessive. That answer depends on the person, but the general answer is: Anything that results in excessive fatigue should be avoided. Also, it's important to note that if there are obvious signs of Kidney deficiency, like premature graying of hair, or a deficiency of Essence, Qi, or Blood, the intervals between bouts of sexual activity should be increased.

Diet: There are many factors to consider when discussing diet's impact on health. Some of these factors, like pesticides and food additives, did not exist in ancient China, but your acupuncturist may discuss them with you. Consumption of genetically modified foods, pesticides, chemicals, flavorings, and food dyes all need to be taken into consideration when looking at the role of the diet in creating disease. Malnutrition is another cause of disease related to diet and can be due to various factors, including poverty, adherence to strict diets, eating disorders, and poor nutritional status in the elderly. Insufficient eating and nutrient intake cause Qi and Blood deficiency and weakens the Spleen, which can kick off a vicious cycle that makes it harder for the Spleen to absorb nutrients from food. Alternatively, overeating can also exhaust the Spleen and Stomach, causing Dampness and Phlegm.

In Chinese medicine, all foods are classified into energetically Hot or Cold categories. Because the Spleen and Stomach prefer warmth, eating too many raw, cold foods (like salads, iced drinks, and ice cream) can damage Stomach Qi. Most acupuncturists, including me, often suggest avoiding excess consumption of raw fruits and vegetables, especially in the winter months. (Soups and stews are a great substitution!) Your acupuncturist may make other suggestions such as steaming your veggies with warming foods like ginger and garlic to make life easier for the Spleen and ditching ice cubes in your winter smoothies (if you must have them) and adding warming spices like cinnamon, clove, and ginger to the blender. When discussing diet with your acupuncturist, you can expect to hear suggestions along these lines.

Lastly, *how* you eat is equally as important as the quality of your food, so your acupuncturist will explore this with you as well. Rushed eating, eating during work, eating too close to bedtime, and eating during emotional distress can all interfere with proper digestion and can injure the Spleen and Stomach.

Chapter Three

Diagnosis and Treatment

IN CHINESE MEDICINE, A SYMPTOM IS JUST A SYMPTOM and can only be understood when the health of the entire body and the relationship of the environment and the emotions are considered. Acupuncturists see each symptom as a puzzle piece, and we need to collect all the pieces to see the whole picture. The holistic nature of Chinese medicine allows us to step back and draw connections that you may not have been aware of. (You might think that your insomnia and your dry skin are totally unrelated, but I don't.)

To get to this broader view of the body, your acupuncturist needs to know very detailed information about your symptoms and your health as a whole. If you come in with a cough, for example, they will want to know whether your cough is dry or phlegmy, whether it is worse at night or during the day, and whether you've also been experiencing digestive issues.

To make a proper diagnosis, your acupuncturist will use the principles discussed in chapter 2 along with the diagnostic methods described in this chapter to create a comprehensive picture of your health. They will then create a treatment plan for you that will help balance the Qi in your body and get you feeling better. In addition, your acupuncturist may also provide a broader plan for how many visits you might need, as well as other lifestyle recommendations.

Characterizing Symptoms

An acupuncturist doesn't just aim to treat an illness by treating your symptoms; they aim to discover and treat the underlying patterns of disharmony in your body that are causing these symptoms. A "pattern" refers to a grouping of symptoms that the acupuncturist will use to make a diagnosis. The acupuncturist determines the pattern by starting with the diagnostic method called the Eight Principles, which, combined with your practitioner's understanding of Qi, Blood, Essence, and Body Fluids as well as the organs, meridians, and the Five Elements, help construct their understanding of your condition.

These Eight Principles—interior, exterior, Hot, Cold, excess, deficiency, Yin, and Yang—provide a very basic foundation for determining a Chinese medicine diagnosis. As your acupuncturist starts to investigate and observe your health, they'll use the Eight Principles to help organize their observations and create a framework that helps interpret the data gathered through the diagnostic methods discussed in the next section. The Eight Principles are separated into four pairs:

Exterior and Interior: *Exterior* and *interior* are used to describe the location of the pattern. Exterior conditions are typically quick in onset and involve symptoms on the surface of the body, like fever and chills, a stiff neck, or a runny nose. Exterior conditions are what conventional Western medicine would refer to as contagious or infectious disease, and they are typically caused by what Chinese medicine calls external pathogens like Cold, Wind, and Dampness. Interior conditions affect internal organs and are usually generated by an imbalance in Qi, like a Spleen Qi deficiency or Liver Qi stagnation.

Hot and Cold: *Hot* and *Cold* describe the general nature and temperature of the pattern. Patterns associated with Hot display signs like redness, inflammation, and hyperactivity of body functions, including rapid pulse, thirst, "jumpiness," and irritability. Patterns associated with Cold display signs like chills, paleness, passiveness, slowness of body functions, and pain that is alleviated by heat.

Excess and Deficiency: *Excess* and *deficiency* are used to describe the strength of the body's Qi as well as the strength of a pathogen. Excess is caused by an external pathogen (like Heat) or caused by stagnations and obstructions of vital substances like Qi, Blood, or Body Fluids, like Liver Heat caused by the stagnation of Liver Qi. Excess often results in feelings of fullness, distention, pressure, and pain. Deficiency is signified by the diminished capacity of an organ or process and results in fatigue, weakness, emptiness, and dull pain that switches locations. In some cases, a pattern can have both excess and deficient aspects—for example, a cold is a combination of an excess external pathogen *and* a deficiency of Wei Qi in the body.

Yin and Yang: These are the broadest of the categories and are used to summarize the three other pairings. Yin characterizes interior, Cold, and deficiency, whereas Yang characterizes exterior, Hot, and excess.

Methods for Diagnosing

Unlike conventional Western medicine, which uses objective measurements like laboratory tests, Chinese medicine diagnosis relies on the perception, skills, and judgment of the practitioner. The four methods of diagnosis are:

- Asking
- Observing
- Listening and smelling
- Palpating (touching or pressing)

These methods become the tools in an acupuncturist's toolbox. To determine your diagnosis, your acupuncturist may use some or all of these methods depending on the situation.

Asking

Your acupuncturist will ask specific questions to help them gather information about all the systems of the body. To assist in this method, Chinese medicine scholars developed the "10 Questions." Inquiring about these 10 subjects will help your acupuncturist discover signs and symptoms you may not necessarily mention up front, thinking that they're not related to your illness.

Temperature: Do you usually feel hot or cold? Do you prefer hot or cold drinks? Is your chief symptom alleviated or aggravated by heat or cold? These questions can help determine if your condition is Hot or Cold, Yin or Yang, and excess or deficient. You may recall from the discussion in chapter 2 on Yin and Yang that you can have excess *true* Heat due to excess Yang, and deficient *false* Heat due to deficient Yin and relative excess Yang.

Sweating: Do you experience night sweats or hot flashes? This might signal a Yin deficiency. Spontaneous sweating without exertion? A possible Qi deficiency. No sweat even during intense workouts? Maybe a Yin or Body Fluids deficiency. Oily sweat? Dampness. This category of questions can help your acupuncturist determine if there are any fluid imbalances in your body and if they are due to excess or deficiency.

Head and Face: Do you have headaches, jaw pain, or sinus congestion? If so, these can all point to underlying imbalances and stagnations. Your acupuncturist will want to know all about the quality of pain and the location—intense forehead headaches might be due to a Stomach imbalance, whereas temple headaches are usually due to a Liver/Gallbladder deficiency. Floaters in the eyes often signify a Blood deficiency, whereas red, bloodshot eyes could be signs of Heat.

Pain: Do you experience any physical pain? Did you have an injury or did the pain appear out of the blue? Is it worse in the morning or night? Is it always in the same spot or does it move around? Is it dull or sharp? What makes it better or worse? Your answers to these questions provide clues about the cause of the pain. Qi stagnation pain tends to travel and be dull, but Blood stagnation pain is usually fixed and throbbing.

Urine and Stools: Do you have a regular daily bowel movement? Congrats, that means your digestive organs are working properly! If you experience constipation, are your bowel movements dry and hard to pass? This could be a Yin deficiency or Heat. Or are they fairly regular but just infrequent? That might be more of a Large Intestine Qi deficiency. If you experience loose stools or diarrhea, do you ever notice undigested food? This means the Spleen isn't "transforming" properly. Does your urinary output match your input? It should! Are you waking up several times a night to urinate? This could be a Kidney imbalance. This might feel like TMI, but body excretions can tell us a lot about our health! It's not uncommon to feel uncomfortable answering these questions, but the answers can be really helpful, so don't be shy.

Thirst and Appetite: Are you always thirsty? This can be Heat or Dryness. Are you thirsty but have no desire to actually drink water? This may signify Heat *with* Dampness or just Dampness. Are you always ravenous? Might be Stomach Heat. No appetite at all and fatigue? Might be a Spleen issue. Cravings for salty foods might be a Kidney deficiency, whereas sweet cravings might point to a Spleen disharmony. Answering specific questions about your thirst, appetite, and cravings can help paint a picture of deeper symptoms in your body.

Sleep: Do you have difficulty falling asleep? This might be a Heart or Shen issue. What about difficulty staying asleep? Or dream-disturbed sleep? Probably a Liver issue. If you frequently wake up at a certain time of night, that may correspond to a specific organ on the Chinese medicine "organ clock"—for example, frequent waking between 1 and 3 a.m. usually points to Liver Qi stagnation, whereas waking between 3 and 5 a.m. points to the Lung.

Chest and Abdomen: Is it hard to take a deep breath? Feeling tightness in your ribs, or rib distention, relates to the Liver, but chest tightness with wheezing relates to the Lungs. Do you have abdominal pain or discomfort? Heartburn might be Stomach Heat, but bloating is probably due to the Spleen. The area and quality of discomfort in the chest and abdomen can help clue your acupuncturist in to specific organ imbalances in your body.

Gynecological (if applicable): How long is your cycle? How many days do you bleed? Is your flow light or heavy? Is the blood brown or bright red? If you have a very light and short flow, with blood that is light in color, that can signify a Blood deficiency. If it is heavy, dark, and clotty, that might mean Blood stagnation. Irregular cycles can be indicative of Yin and Yang imbalances. Again, this can sometimes be embarrassing to talk about, but often symptoms that women consider "normal" can actually be important signals that point to underlying issues.

Lifestyle and Habits: What do you eat? How often do you exercise? How often do you drink alcohol? Do you struggle with any particular emotions? How is your parents' health? Your acupuncturist will probably want to know about your lifestyle and habits, including your typical diet, your activity level, and overall emotional well-being. They will also want to know about family history and any other factors that might impact your health.

Observing

Your acupuncturist will observe your general appearance, complexion, and tongue for other "clues." Redness in the face, for example, can indicate Heat, and a pale face can indicate Cold or a Blood deficiency. Dry hair, nails, and skin can indicate a Yin deficiency, and conversely, a swollen, puffy face can indicate Dampness. Your stature and body type can also provide insight into your constitutional tendencies, which might predispose you to certain imbalances. A thin and wiry body is more Yang and might be more likely to experience Yin deficiency, whereas a plumper, rounder body is more Yin and more likely to experience Dampness. While your acupuncturist won't make a diagnosis based *just* on your appearance and body type, it does provide some clues to what might be going on.

Observation of the tongue, called tongue diagnosis, is an integral part of Chinese medicine. Your acupuncturist can discern a surprising amount of information about your health from the shape, color, and coating of your tongue. A healthy tongue is pale red, slightly moist, and evenly shaped with a thin white "fur." A pale, swollen tongue with "scallop" tooth marks can indicate a Qi deficiency, whereas a cherry-red tongue indicates Heat. If only a certain area of the tongue is red, it can signify Heat in the corresponding organ on the tongue map (see page 48).

Someone with Heart Heat and symptoms like anxiety, insomnia, or overthinking will typically have a red tip on their tongue. People with chronic asthma or Lung deficiency often have a little dip in the Lung region. Liver Qi stagnation, with signs like irritability and PMS, often appears as an orange or red tone and pinching or scallops on the edges of the tongue. A purple quality to the tongue can indicate Cold or Blood stagnation.

Tongue coating is related to the health of Body Fluids. A shiny tongue with no coat at all can signify a Body Fluids deficiency, whereas a tongue with a thick, greasy coating can signify Dampness. If the tongue coating is yellow, it can signify Heat. But keep in mind that certain foods and medications can also affect your tongue—coffee, for example, will turn your tongue coating yellow and Pepto-Bismol will turn it black—so this is never used as the *only* method of diagnosis.

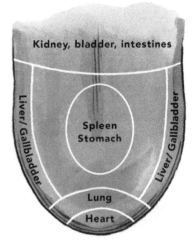

Listening and Smelling

Thanks to modern hygiene, smelling is no longer a major part of diagnosis, but certain body smells can indicate imbalances. Bad breath can often be linked to Stomach Heat, and sour body odor can be related to Damp-Heat. Listening to the quality of the voice and breath can also help identify an imbalance, so your acupuncturist may take note of things like weak voice or shallow/wheezy breathing.

Pulse Palpating

Pulse palpation is another important diagnos the pulse at three different locations on each wrist (as shown in the illustration on the right), your acupuncturist can tell a lot about the quality of Qi and Blood in your body as it relates to specific organs.

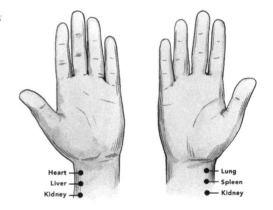

A normal, healthy pulse flows smoothly and consistently through the arteries. Each of the three pulse areas on each wrist relate to specific organs, and organ imbalances can often be felt in the pulse. The classical texts discuss 28 types of pulses. Each type—with names like "choppy," "wiry," and "slippery"—considers the depth, speed, width, and strength of the pulse and can each signify a different imbalance. For example, a "choppy" pulse indicates Blood stagnation, whereas a "wiry" pulse indicates Liver Qi stagnation, and a "slippery" pulse indicates Dampness. A "floating" pulse, where the pulse is felt when barely touching the skin, indicates that the Wei Qi is active; you might either already be sick or feel like you're coming down with something.

It takes a lot of time and experience to feel these subtle differences in the pulse, but an adept practitioner can ascertain a lot of information about your overall health using pulse palpation.

Creating a Treatment Plan

Each point on the body has a specific function for its meridian or organ. There are about 365 main acupuncture points, not including several dozen "extra" points. It's up to your acupuncturist to choose exactly which points to use to create the point prescription—many points have similar functions and effects. Choosing between these is what makes every acupuncturist and every treatment different, and this is where the "art" of acupuncture lies.

A proper diagnosis does more than identify a grouping of symptoms; it also helps define the therapeutic principles. If Qi is stuck, the treatment principle will be to move Qi. If Blood is deficient, the treatment principle will be to nourish Blood. If the Shen is disturbed, the treatment principle will be to calm the Shen. Determining the treatment principle then allows your acupuncturist to choose points that have the intended effect. For example, if you have signs of Liver Qi stagnation with headaches and irritability, they will pick points that help move Liver Qi, soothe the Liver, and calm the Shen. Your treatment may also include the use of moxibustion, cupping, or gua sha. Some acupuncturists might also prescribe herbs.

Everyone responds to acupuncture differently, so it's not easy to say *exactly* how many treatments you will need, but based on your acupuncturist's knowledge and experience, they will tell you how many treatments they expect you might need or how many you'll want before reevaluating to see if acupuncture works for you. This is called the treatment plan. The general rule of thumb is that the longer you've had the issue, the longer it might take to see progress. Your treatment plan might also include dietary or lifestyle recommendations based on your diagnosis.

In the Office

After reviewing your health history in depth, your acupuncturist will get you ready for your treatment. Most acupuncturists use massage tables and will have you lie either faceup or facedown depending on the points they plan to use. They will make sure you are resting comfortably and that the skin is exposed in the area they plan to needle.

For most treatments, you can keep on any clothing covering areas that won't be needled (that is, receive needle insertion). Because the most commonly used acupuncture points are found below the knees and elbows, it's always a good idea to wear clothing that allows your acupuncturist access to those areas. (Acupuncturists often joke about skinny jeans being the worst thing that happens at their office because they usually need to be removed!) If you do need to take clothing off, your acupuncturist will use sheets or towels to cover areas that don't require needling.

Your acupuncturist might swab the points they plan to use with alcohol. This is only necessary if a point is visibly dirty, but it used to be the health code, so many acupuncturists still do it out of habit. Next, they will begin needle insertion. If you are new to acupuncture and feeling anxious, they may coach you on breathing techniques while inserting the needles to help you relax. Needling happens very quickly, and it's not uncommon for me to hear a surprised "Wait, that's it?! I expected it to be way worse!" at the end of someone's first needling experience. (See, I told you it's not as scary as it sounds!)

You will then rest with the needles in place for about 20 to 40 minutes. According to the classical texts, it takes about 28 minutes for Qi to circulate one time through the body, so I like to leave needles in for at least that long, but sometimes I leave them in for up to 45 minutes, especially for my patients who like to take a solid "acu-nap." Depending on the office setup, your acupuncturist may stay in the room with you or may leave to take care of other patients while you rest. I give my patients a bell they can ring if they need me. Because of acupuncture's ability to help you relax, most people fall asleep or find themselves in a very restful state during this time.

At the end of the treatment, your acupuncturist will remove the needles and might perform adjunctive techniques like moxibustion, gua sha, or cupping. If these techniques are going to be used, your acupuncturist will discuss this with you beforehand.

At your next visit, you will review any changes since your last treatment and discuss any new issues that may have arisen. The points your acupuncturist uses may change from session to session based on several factors, including your progress and any new issues that may have arisen.

A Closer Look at Acupuncture Treatment

So, now that you know how acupuncturists make their diagnoses and what to expect once you're in the office, you might be wondering what exactly is going on during that period of time when your acupuncturist is sticking needles in you! In the upcoming section, you'll learn a bit about what acupuncture points are and how your acupuncturist decides which points to use for you.

What Are Points?

Each meridian has a set number of named by the meridian's organ and the order of the points on the meridian, but they each also have a descriptive name that describes the point's characteristic or location. Stomach 1, for example, located just below the pupil, is called "Tear Container," and Bladder 1, located at the inner corner of the eye, is called "Bright Eyes." This illustration of the acupuncture meridians and points on the head can help you visualize this a little better.

The number of points on each meridian ranges from 9 (for the Pericardium meridian) to 67 (for the Urinary Bladder meridian). There are 365 regular points

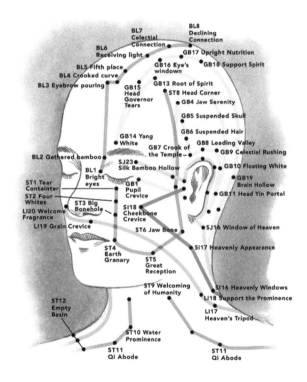

to choose from and dozens of "extra" points. Each point has specific indications and functions. And, yes, acupuncturists have to memorize them all, including the functions, indications, needling angles, and safe needling depths. Acupuncture school, you may have guessed, is no joke. And while you don't *really* need to know the following information (unless you're in acupuncture school), it should help provide some context for why certain points are used more frequently than others.

In daily practice, there are fewer than 100 points that are most commonly used by most acupuncturists—these points are the most effective for treating a variety of issues. But 100 is still a lot, so with all of these possible points to choose from, and with most treatments consisting of 8 to 20 needles, how does an acupuncturist decide which points to use?

Your acupuncturist will probably use a combination of local and distal points. Local points are ones that lie near or over the area of concern—for example, we'll use abdominal points for diarrhea, knee points for knee pain, and points near the nose for congestion. Distal points are ones farther away from the area of concern but are usually located on the affected meridian. To narrow down which points to use, we use a system of point categories that groups together points on each meridian with similar effects and functions.

The "transporting points," one of the most important categories of points, describe how Qi is transported through the meridians. Each meridian has a Jing-Well, Ying-Spring, Shu-Stream, Jing-River, and He-Sea point. The Jing-Well point is always the first or last point on a meridian, located at the tip of a finger or toe, whereas the Qi is thought to "bubble"—these points are often used to settle the Shen, whereas the He-Sea points, usually found near the elbow or knee, play a role in settling the digestive system.

Each meridian also has a Yuan-source point where the Qi can be most easily activated, a Xi-cleft point where the Qi and Blood come together that can be useful for pain, and a Luo-connecting point where each meridian diverges to meet its pair, allowing for the ability to treat more than one meridian with a single point. Points that belong to these categories are typically the most effective and most commonly used of all the points during an acupuncture treatment.

We also have "influential points" that have specific symptoms and areas that they treat, and "alarm points" whose tenderness can indicate an imbalance. For example, Ren 17 on the chest is the influential point of Qi, and Gallbladder 34 near the knee is the influential point of tendons. Lung 1 is the alarm point of the Lungs, and tenderness at this point, near the area where the collarbone and arm meet, can signify Lung issues. There are also specific points that have the function of clearing the external pathogens from the body. Gallbladder 20, where the back of the skull and neck meet, can clear Wind, whereas Large Intestine 11, at the outer crease of the elbow, clears Heat.

We also sometimes use points that aren't on a specific meridian but correlate to an area of pain. Tender points are called ah-shi points (sometimes also called trigger points) and are needled to disperse Qi and reduce pain in the local area.

And that's not all . . . because each of the main meridians exists on both the right and left sides of the body, your acupuncturist also has to decide if they will choose a point on both sides or just one. (This is a matter of preference. There are certain points that I almost always use on both sides, and there are others that I typically use on just one side and pair with a similar point on the opposite side.)

All of these point categories help provide the structure on which your acupuncturist will base your treatment plan and point prescription.

Locating Points

Once your acupuncturist has decided which points to use, how do they find them on your body? Acupuncture point location is based on a unit of measurement called a cun (pronounced *tsoon*), or body inch. As everyone's body is different, cun measurements are proportional to each person and are not fixed amounts. The width of every person's thumb, regardless of actual size, is one cun; the width of the other four fingers as a group is three cun (see the illustration below). Each limb and area of the body has a specific cun measurement.

For example, the length from the outer crease of the elbow to the area where the wrist meets the thumb is 12 cun. The cun on the arm of a baby will be much smaller than that of a grown man, but both arms are 12 cun. Acupuncture point locations are all described using a combination of these measurements, other acupuncture points, and anatomical features. Here are two examples:

- The point Spleen 6 is located three cun above the inner ankle bone, just behind the tibia.
- Lung 6 is located on the forearm, on the line joining Lung 9 and Lung 5, seven cun above the wrist crease.

Acupuncturists learn several ways of measuring to find the location of the point. If I am treating a patient whose hands and body are about the size of my own, I use the

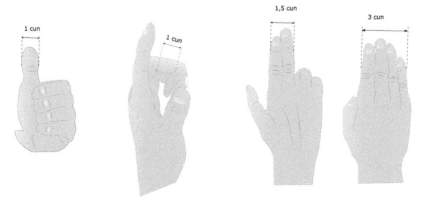

width of my own thumb and fingers to help locate the points. If I am treating someone who is much larger or smaller than I am, I break down their bodies into the cun measurements. For example, if I'm trying to locate a point that's three cun below the knee, and I know that the lower leg is 12 cun long, I'll visualize and use my hands to approximate a quarter of the way down the leg.

Learning to memorize, measure, and locate points is an essential part of acupuncture training, and proper point location requires knowledge of the body measurements, palpation skills, and a good heap of judgment.

Needling Techniques

There is much more to needling than just poking a needle into the skin. Proper needle technique can take a long time to master. Long before they can needle a patient, acupuncture students practice their needle techniques on bars of soap, small oranges, and each other. Painless insertion requires being both quick and gentle. Each point has a very specific needling angle and depth that an acupuncturist must know to efficiently activate Qi and also to prevent injury to surrounding tissues and organs. Depending on the area of the body, the Qi is located at different depths. Qi on the hands and feet is right at the surface, so the needles are barely inserted through the upper layer of skin. Qi in the larger muscles is located deeper and activation requires deeper needle insertion.

There are several ways to activate Qi, and different needle techniques are used based on what the intended goal is. Some needle techniques help reinforce or strengthen Qi, while others help reduce or disperse Qi. While there are other variations of needle technique, such as clockwise and counterclockwise twisting, these are the most common:

> **Lifting and thrusting**: To reinforce Qi, the needle is inserted with a quick and heavy thrust, and lifted gently and slowly. To reduce or disperse Qi, the needle is inserted gently and slowly, and lifted quickly and forcefully.

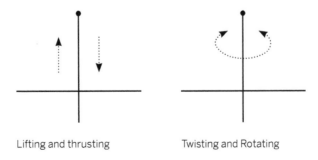

Lifting and thrusting   Twisting and Rotating

Twisting and rotating: To reinforce Qi, the needle is twisted and rotated slowly; to reduce or disperse Qi, the needle is twisted and rotated quickly.

Why Doesn't It Hurt?

When we conjure up an image of a needle, we are typically thinking of the type of needle used for injections and drawing blood. These needles are thick and hollow, allowing for fluid or blood to pass through the center. Acupuncture needles, on the other hand, are hair-thin and solid. In fact, acupuncture needles are so thin that, depending on the gauge, or width, of the needles, several acupuncture needles can fit in the tip of one syringe.

Acupuncturists may use different length and gauge needles (or pins as we sometimes call them) depending on their personal preference and the area of the body they're needling, but all acupuncture needles are typically painless. This doesn't mean, however, that you won't feel the needle (it's not invisible!), but the sensation is usually more of a dull ache or slight tingle.

Because the needles are so thin, many acupuncturists use guide tubes that help ensure a smooth, gentle, and quick insertion into the skin. Upon insertion, your acupuncturist may try to elicit de Qi ("grabbing of the Qi") using some of the needle techniques described earlier. You may experience this as a sensation of pulling or throbbing at the point, and it is a sign that Qi has been activated. Many patients come to enjoy and even look forward to this sensation. Acupuncturists can feel the "grab," too! Classical Chinese Medicine texts describe this feeling as similar to what a person fishing feels when a fish gets hooked on a fishing line, and after experiencing this sensation many thousands of times, I can say it's still the most accurate description I've read.

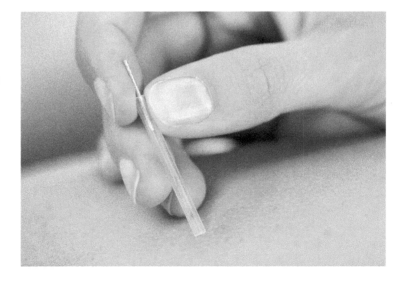

Part Two

Common Ailments in the Office

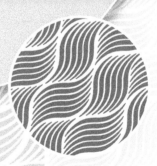

Chapter Four

Acupuncture in Action

WELCOME TO THE OFFICE! THIS CHAPTER includes descriptions of 20 different ailments commonly treated by acupuncturists. Of course, this is just a sampling of the many conditions that acupuncture can help. For each ailment, I'll discuss typical patterns that may be causing symptoms, as well as potential treatments. This can give you an idea of what it's like to be a real patient.

Keep in mind that every acupuncturist is different, using their own methods and techniques to diagnose and treat a patient. To explain this, I often use the analogy of a Rubik's Cube: There are a lot of correct ways to turn the pieces to solve the puzzle. Remember also that acupuncturists treat people—not illnesses. These examples are meant to give you an idea of how we think about certain conditions, but this chapter simplifies diagnosis and just scratches the surface of what we might think about. Seek out the advice of a licensed acupuncturist to receive an accurate diagnosis and customized plan.

Managing Expectations

Acupuncture is built on the principle that every body is different. Two people may be affected by Wind-Cold, but the person with the stronger Qi may experience a briefer or milder illness. Liver Qi stagnation might cause pain in one person but irritability and insomnia in the next. A Kidney Qi deficiency could manifest as chronic low back pain in one person but premature graying hair in someone else. And because we are all unique, it can be hard to know at the first visit how many treatments your condition will require.

Because this is "slow" medicine, you can almost always expect to require several visits before experiencing lasting change. I do, however, always hope to see some signs of improvement after the first visit. Sometimes these improvements aren't related to the chief symptom but involve other areas, like sleep or digestion. These kinds of things help me recognize that we are on the right track. At each visit, I will ask patients about symptoms they previously reported, and I often find that patients don't notice improvements until I ask about them. For example, I might ask, "How have your headaches been this week?" And they may respond, "I hadn't even realized, but I don't think I've had one!" Scholars call this negativity bias—we are way more likely to notice the things that are wrong than we are to notice positive improvements.

Just like with medication, acupuncture dosage is important. Saying, "I tried acupuncture once and it didn't work" is a lot like saying, "I went to the gym once and didn't feel stronger." Effects are cumulative, so if you're going to give acupuncture a try, stick with it for a little while before judging if it works for you! I recommend scheduling your first few appointments as close together as possible, as each treatment builds on the last. It's also important to be open to lifestyle recommendations that your acupuncturist makes; these can often have a huge impact on the speed of recovery. For example, if you suffer from bloating and indigestion, removing cold and raw foods from your diet, along with regular acupuncture, will give you much quicker results than with just acupuncture alone.

The relationship between an acupuncturist and a patient is more of a partnership than anything else. I like to tell patients that they are in charge of their healing—I'm just the guide to show them (and their bodies) the way. Now let's look at some of the most common ailments seen in acupuncture clinics.

Acne

In Chinese medicine, acne, despite being a condition on the surface of the body, is always a sign of an underlying imbalance. As much as we'd like to believe that acne is left behind with all the other awkward growing pains of adolescence, acne can continue to plague some people through adulthood. Western dermatology tends to focus primarily on symptom management, with medications used to treat the local inflammation. There isn't always emphasis on finding out why the inflammation is happening in the first place, which is where Chinese medicine excels.

Acne is differentiated in Chinese medicine by what the pimples look like. Red, inflamed pimples are a sign of toxic Heat in the Blood, whereas pale, cystic (fluid-filled) pimples are a sign of Dampness. Red and cystic acne is a combination of the two; we call this Damp-Heat. The cause of toxic Heat is usually related to diet or emotions, so your acupuncturist will probably focus their questions on those two areas. Dark red/almost purple acne can be related to Blood stagnation in the body and is usually accompanied by other signs of this pattern like heavy, clotty periods in women. Treating acne from the root cause can take longer than going the conventional medication route, but healing it this way can have dramatic effects without the potentially harmful side effects of pharmaceutical treatment.

Diagnosis and Treatment

The primary patterns we look for when treating acne are:

Toxic Heat: Red, inflamed pimples that might be painful; worsens with spicy food or alcohol

Dampness: Cystic, pus-filled acne; worsens with dairy and sugar; accompanies other signs of Dampness like fatigue and diarrhea

Damp-Heat: Combination of red and cystic acne

Blood Stagnation: Dark red/purple pimples accompanied by heavy, clotty periods; may worsen the week before menstruation

Acne is one of the best examples of root and branch diagnosis in Chinese medicine. Acne, while appearing on the skin, is very rarely *just* a skin issue. Clearing up chronic acne requires looking at why it is occurring in the first place. Acne treatments are usually combined with dietary recommendations, especially removing Damp- and Heat-producing foods like dairy, sugar, spicy foods, and alcohol from the diet. If your acne tends to be worse before your period, getting regular acupuncture and especially focusing on the week before your symptoms arise can be very helpful.

Allergies

In Chinese medicine, seasonal allergies always relate to a deficiency in your Wei Qi, which protects the exterior of the body. This Qi deficiency allows external pathogens to enter the body and can be caused by several organ imbalances. The specific allergy symptoms help clue us in to which organ is off. The Lungs are almost always implicated, as they are in charge of the Wei Qi, but they also control the nose and throat, so the most common symptoms of allergies such as a scratchy throat, runny nose, and sneezing all point to a Lung disharmony.

Certain symptoms also point to the specific external pathogens that may have invaded the body; itchiness is caused by Wind, while redness of the eyes and nose might be due to Heat. Acupuncture can be helpful in treating symptoms of allergies when they appear, but it's best at preventing allergy symptoms before they start. If you typically get spring or fall allergies, it's ideal to start receiving regular weekly acupuncture at least one to two months before your symptoms typically start.

Diagnosis and Treatment

The primary patterns we look for when treating allergies are:

Wei Qi/Lung Qi Deficiency: Allergies, catching colds easily, wheezing and sneezing

Wind-Cold: Acute-onset allergies, with itchiness and chills

Wind-Heat: Acute-onset allergies, with redness and thick, yellow mucus and red eyes

Preventing seasonal allergies before they flare up is much easier than treating symptoms once they've started, so planning ahead is key. By working to support your Wei Qi, acupuncture is very effective in keeping your body strong to prevent symptoms. If you're already experiencing allergy symptoms, acupuncture can help open and clear the sinuses, reduce headaches, and decrease inflammation in the respiratory tract. There are also several classical Chinese herbal formulas that help alleviate allergy symptoms without the side effects that antihistamines can cause, like drowsiness and dry mouth, so if your acupuncturist is also an herbalist, they might prescribe you herbs.

Anxiety

Anxiety is one of the most common issues that brings people into an acupuncturist's office. Occasional anxiety is actually a very normal response to stressful or new situations, and if you've ever taken final exams or gone on a first date, you've probably experienced it. However, for some people, this feeling of fear and worry can become chronic and interfere with their daily lives, even manifesting in debilitating panic and anxiety attacks. Acupuncture can be used in addition to, or as a safe and effective alternative to, medication. Research backs this up: Scientists believe that acupuncture helps regulate neurotransmitters and increase levels of our feel-good chemicals called endorphins. Several clinical trials have found acupuncture to be a very effective treatment for generalized anxiety and panic disorders, with few side effects compared to conventional treatment.

In Chinese medicine, anxiety is defined as a disturbance of the Shen and can have several root causes. By asking you various questions about your symptoms and the manifestation of your anxiety, as well as asking about other things going on in your body, your acupuncturist will determine where your imbalance is and treat your anxiety from the root, while also using points known to help settle the Shen.

Diagnosis and Treatment

The primary patterns we look for when treating anxiety are:

Liver Qi Stagnation: Anxiety, PMS, irritability, rib tenderness, cold hands and feet, and insomnia with difficulty staying asleep or waking up between 1 and 3 a.m.

Liver Heat: Anxiety with a temper, headaches, and a red complexion

Heart Blood Deficiency: Anxiety along with insomnia or difficulty falling asleep, palpitations, pale skin and lips, poor memory, and light periods in women

Yin Deficiency: Anxiety, night sweats, restlessness, and thirst; a common pattern during menopause

Your acupuncturist will most likely use points that are known to calm the Shen along with points to treat the root pattern. They may also provide other recommendations such as herbal formulas, dietary modifications, and gentle exercises like yoga and qigong. While most people feel a reduction in anxiety after their first treatment, it may take several treatments to feel a lasting effect. I typically recommend weekly treatments for four to six weeks, or until anxiety symptoms feel more manageable.

DIY Acupressure: Anxiety

The following acupressure points can be used to calm the Shen, no matter the root cause. Using your fingertips, apply moderate pressure for 60 to 90 seconds in a circular motion while taking deep, restorative breaths. Do this as often as needed when experiencing anxiety symptoms.

YIN TANG

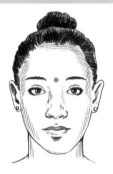

Located above the bridge of the nose between the eyebrows.

This point helps calm the spirit and focus the mind.

SHEN MEN

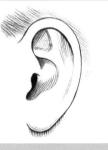

Located in the triangular fossa in the ear.

This point promotes relaxation and healing.

KIDNEY 1

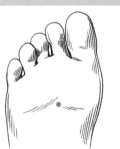

Located at the depression in the foot when the toes are pointed.

This is one of the most grounding points on the body and can help settle the mind.

Arthritis

Arthritis is defined as painful inflammation and stiffness in the joints. There are several different types of arthritis. Osteoarthritis (OA) is the most common form and includes symptoms like pain, swelling, stiffness, and decreased range of motion in one or several joints. Osteoarthritis is caused by degeneration of cartilage between the bones due to age or overuse and is typically diagnosed based on symptoms and with X-ray imaging. Rheumatoid arthritis (RA) is an autoimmune condition that causes inflammation of the tissues that cushion the joints.

Western medical treatment for arthritis often includes the use of steroid medications that can have several unpleasant side effects, so many arthritis sufferers turn to acupuncture for relief—and for good reason! Acupuncture has provided relief from arthritis pain for centuries, and modern-day research backs up its safety and efficacy.

In Chinese medicine, arthritic pain is referred to as Bi Syndrome. It is caused by a stagnation of Qi and Blood, which can be due to external pathogens becoming trapped in the meridians. To restore proper Qi and Blood flow, and clear any obstructions, it may take several treatments before feeling relief. I typically recommend six to eight weekly acupuncture treatments before evaluating if acupuncture is helping relieve your pain and stiffness.

Diagnosis and Treatment

There are many different patterns attributed to Bi Syndrome. Common patterns include:

Wind Predominant: Traveling pain and stiffness

Cold Predominant: Severe pain with fixed location with sensation of cold; aggravated by cold weather and alleviated by warmth

Dampness Predominant: Heavy feeling in the joints with swelling and numbness; worse on rainy and humid days

Heat Predominant: Local redness, swelling, and burning sensation; aggravated by hot and humid weather; may be warm to the touch

Blood Stagnation: Chronic long-term pain, often with deformity of joints

Qi Stagnation: Pain that comes and goes, often due to overuse of a joint

It is common to see combinations of these patterns, such as Wind-Damp-Cold and Wind-Damp-Heat.

Your acupuncturist will most likely use points that are local to the area of pain to disperse Qi and Blood, while also using points elsewhere on the affected meridians to encourage proper flow. If you have a Cold-predominant type of arthritis, your acupuncturist might also apply heat or use moxibustion, which can warm the joint. We generally don't encourage using ice in Chinese medicine, as it can cause stagnation and slow down healing, so if your arthritis is more of a Heat type, your acupuncturist will likely use points to clear Heat and support the Yin (cooling aspect) of the body.

Because of the inflammatory nature of all types of arthritis, your acupuncturist may include dietary recommendations, like limiting greasy, fatty, and Damp-producing foods such as fried food and dairy, which can contribute to Dampness and stagnation in the body. To encourage proper Qi and Blood flow, your acupuncturist may encourage gentle exercise like yoga or tai chi.

Back Pain

Back pain affects most adults at some point in their lives. Back pain manifests in a variety of ways; it can be a dull, inconsistent ache; a traveling, nervy pain; or a sharp, debilitating pain. It's the second-most prevalent reason for a person to visit a doctor in the United States and one of the leading causes of missing work. Simply put, back pain is a huge pain in the rear!

In Chinese medicine we categorize back pain based on the afflicted meridian as well as the quality and intensity of pain. An acute back injury is typically a stagnation of Qi or Blood, whereas chronic low back pain is typically a Kidney Qi deficiency. Sciatica, a type of chronic back pain characterized by radiating pain beginning in the low back and extending down the legs, is often a combination of local Qi and Blood stagnation with a Kidney deficiency and/or Cold-Damp in the meridians.

By using a combination of local and distal points, acupuncture is incredibly successful in treating back pain. A German study in 2007 found that acupuncture was twice as effective for treating low back pain than conventional therapies, including pain relievers and physical therapy.

DIY Acupressure: Back Pain

The following acupressure points are often used in the treatment of low back pain. Using your fingertips, apply moderate pressure to these points for 60 to 90 seconds in a circular motion on the affected side or both sides if pain travels or occurs on both sides. Do this several times a day, as needed.

LARGE INTESTINE 4

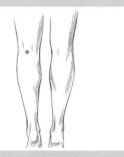

Located in the meaty part of the hand between the thumb and forefinger.

This point helps move Qi anywhere in the body and is great for all types of pain.

URINARY BLADDER 40

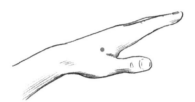

Located in the back of the knee at the center of the crease.

This point is known as the lumbar command point and is helpful for all low back pain.

GALLBLADDER 30

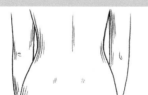

Located on the buttocks one-third of the way between the head of the femur bone and the tailbone.

This point resolves pain in the hip region and is usually tender to the touch. It's especially helpful for sciatica.

Diagnosis and Treatment

The primary patterns we look for when treating back pain are:

Kidney Qi Deficiency: Chronic, achy, dull low back pain, sometimes accompanied by knee pain; may also be accompanied by premature graying of hair or dental issues

Blood Stagnation: Acute, intense pain, usually caused by a trauma; worsens with pressure

Qi Stagnation: Pain that switches sides, chronic, but not debilitating; worse with stress

Damp-Cold Invasion: Sciatica and other hip and low back pain that is worse on cold or damp days

Depending on the pattern of disharmony, your acupuncturist will choose a series of local and distal points to move Qi and Blood in the meridians and reduce pain. There are several distal points known for their ability to treat back pain of any cause, and your acupuncturist will probably use some of these points in your treatment. (See "DIY Acupressure: Back Pain" on page 67 to try these for yourself!) Acute back pain may take only a few treatments to get the Qi and Blood moving again, whereas chronic back pain may take several consecutive treatments to focus on the root imbalances.

Acupuncturists often also use heat, moxibustion, cupping, or gua sha to treat back pain. They may also recommend applying heat at home, taking hot baths to promote blood flow through the muscles, and making changes in sitting or driving postures to help alleviate and prevent pain.

Colds and Flus

In Chinese medicine, colds and flus result from an external pathogen invading the body. Whether or not you get sick is a result of two factors: the strength of that external pathogen and the strength of your body's protective Wei Qi. Because acupuncture helps regulate and support Qi, regular acupuncture treatments can be very helpful in preventing illnesses like this. If you do come down with a cold or flu, acupuncture can help clear the external pathogens and build the Wei Qi to reduce the length and severity of the illness and lessen discomfort. Studies have shown that acupuncture helps activate the body's T cells, which are important immune-system regulators.

DIY Acupressure: Common Cold

The following acupressure points can be very helpful in clearing congestion, easing coughing, and resolving headaches while fighting a cold. Using your fingertips, apply moderate pressure to each point for 60 to 90 seconds in a circular motion while taking deep, restorative breaths. Do this several times a day to relieve cold symptoms.

YIN TANG

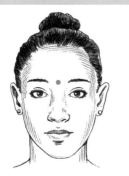

Located above the bridge of the nose between the eyebrows.

This point moves Qi in the head and is great for nasal congestion.

LARGE INTESTINE 4

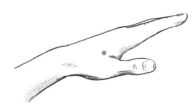

Located in the meaty part of the hand between the thumb and forefinger.

This is the command point of the front of the head and is great for headaches, sinus congestion, and sneezing.

REN 17

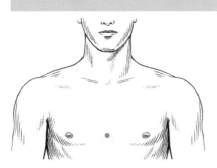

Located on the sternum (breastbone) directly between the nipples.

This point regulates Lung Qi and helps open the chest, making breathing easier.

Diagnosis and Treatment

The primary patterns we look for when treating colds and flus are:

Wind-Cold Invasion: Any or all of the following: Subjective feeling of cold with aversion to cold; chills more predominant than fever; headaches starting at the back of the head; sneezing; clear, profuse phlegm

Wind-Heat Invasion: Any or all of the following: subjective feeling of heat with aversion to heat; fever more predominant than chills; sore throat; agitation; yellow phlegm; red eyes

Colds and flus usually need to run their course, but acupuncture can be helpful in keeping your immune system strong and preventing you from getting sick in the first place. If you do get sick but feel well enough to leave your house, getting in to see your acupuncturist can reduce the length and severity of your illness. Don't worry about getting us sick—acupuncturists tend to have pretty strong immune systems!

Depression

As discussed in chapter 2, in Chinese medicine, emotions are intimately connected to the organs and contribute to overall balance in the body. Sadness, grief, fear, and anger are all considered normal emotions until they become out of balance with or more prevalent than the other emotions. Symptoms of depression like apathy, melancholy, fatigue, and body pain all point to an underlying imbalance in the Qi and Blood and are often tied to the Liver and Heart, the two organs that have the largest roles in dealing with emotions.

Depression is complex and can manifest in many different ways and for many different causes. In Chinese medicine we identify types of depression by whether the symptoms are *excess* or *deficient* (page 27). Excess signs of depression include chest distention, pain, and anger, whereas deficient signs of depression include fatigue, lethargy, and apathy.

Diagnosis and Treatment

The primary patterns we look for when treating depression are:

Liver Qi Stagnation: Depression, irritability, PMS, inability to take a deep breath, rib tightness

Phlegm-Dampness: Depression, heaviness, feeling of "pit" in throat

Heart Blood Deficiency: Depression, dizziness, pallor, fatigue, amenorrhea, palpitations; a common pattern in postpartum depression

Lung Qi Deficiency: Prolonged grief that doesn't resolve after loss; may also accompany shallow breathing or difficulty taking a deep breath

All emotional conditions in Chinese medicine are tied to the Shen, so your acupuncturist will typically use points that are known to help calm and soothe the Shen. They will also use points to treat your specific underlying pattern. Because of acupuncture's direct effect on neurotransmitters (see chapter 1 for more information), many patients feel an immediate improvement in mood following acupuncture. How long these effects last can differ from patient to patient, but regular acupuncture can be very effective in reducing depressive symptoms and contributing to an overall healthy mood.

If you notice that winter seems to be especially difficult for you (this is called seasonal affective disorder; SAD), receiving regular acupuncture in the weeks leading up to and through winter can help lessen the impact of seasonal change. Modern research has found acupuncture to be an effective treatment for depression, both in place of and in combination with antidepressant medications, and acupuncture can often help lessen the side effects that patients on antidepressant medications experience. Always speak with your doctor before making any changes to prescribed medications.

Fertility

Acupuncture can help balance hormones, regulate cycles, increase egg quality, prevent miscarriage, and support a healthy pregnancy, making it useful for women with a range of infertility issues.

By using acupuncture points on the meridians to treat underlying imbalances as well as local points on the abdomen to stimulate blood flow to the reproductive organs, acupuncture has earned a well-deserved reputation for helping many women get pregnant. In fact, a lot of ob-gyns, despite not knowing exactly *how* it works, recommend acupuncture to their patients before sending them to a fertility specialist. And because of its effectiveness, fertility specialists also often recommend that patients undergoing fertility treatments also receive acupuncture. Studies have shown that acupuncture in conjunction with in vitro fertilization (IVF) increases the chance of a viable pregnancy.

And since it takes two to tango, we can't forget to mention sperm quality. Male infertility issues related to sperm count and motility (ability to "swim") are on the rise and becoming a major part of the infertility landscape. Studies suggest that acupuncture can also be used to help increase sperm quality in men.

Diagnosis and Treatment

The primary patterns we look for when treating issues with fertility:

Kidney Yin Deficiency: Shorter follicular phase, high follicle-stimulating hormone (FSH), low estrogen, night sweats

Kidney Yang Deficiency: Shorter luteal phase, low progesterone, feeling cold frequently

Liver Qi Stagnation: Stress, irritability, PMS, cold hands and feet

Blood Stagnation: Clotty, painful, heavy periods

Blood Deficiency: Amenorrhea or irregular periods, fatigue, pale skin, and lips; patient might have iron-deficiency anemia

Because of acupuncture's popularity among women trying to get pregnant, many acupuncturists specialize in fertility and have practices that are dedicated, solely or in part, to working with this population. A large portion of my practice is working with women experiencing fertility challenges, and getting their "I'm pregnant!" emails (and sometimes photos of just-peed-on pregnancy tests) is one of the most joyous and gratifying parts of my job. As the struggle to get pregnant is typically filled with stress and anxiety, the emotional healing that acupuncture offers can be an added benefit during this time.

Depending on your pattern diagnosis, your acupuncturist will recommend a treatment frequency that might range from twice a week to twice a month. For patients hoping to get pregnant naturally, I typically suggest getting regular acupuncture for at least three to four months to see if it can help. When patients are going through in vitro fertilization, I like to work with them during the stimulation and retrieval phase, and then in the week leading up to and just after the embryo transfer. Once we get what is known in the fertility world as the BFP (Big Fat Positive, aka positive pregnancy test), we move on to supporting the pregnancy and preventing and treating some of the known issues that occur during this very exciting time. See also "Pregnancy" on page 83.

Headaches and Migraines

It's hard to find an adult who has never had a headache! Hormone imbalance, food sensitivities, dehydration, tight neck and shoulder muscles, and stress can all trigger headaches. For some people with chronic headaches, the exact cause is frustratingly unknown. Chronic headaches and migraines can be debilitating for many people, and pharmaceutical treatment isn't always effective and can have some unwanted side effects. Pain is one of the instances in Chinese medicine where we aim to treat both the root *and* the branch, trying to alleviate the symptoms as quickly as possible and working to correct the root imbalance causing them. Studies suggest that acupuncture can effectively reduce the severity and frequency of migraines and tension-type headaches.

In conventional Western medicine, headaches are categorized into groups like cluster, tension, sinus, and migraine. In Chinese medicine, we focus on the area of the head and the meridian where the headaches are experienced. Frontal headaches are often related to the Stomach organ and meridian, occipital headaches are related to the Kidneys and Urinary Bladder, and temple headaches are related to the Gallbladder. Just like in conventional Western medicine, there are numerous possible causes of headaches and lots of contributing factors, so your acupuncturist will do a very thorough intake interview to help figure out all of the puzzle pieces.

Diagnosis and Treatment

There are dozens of possible patterns for headaches, and pattern diagnosis depends on where the headaches are experienced, how frequently, and what makes them better or worse. It's easiest to break down headaches into categories of external and internal causes.

External: Headaches can be caused by any of the external pathogens (see page 38). These are usually quick-onset and short-duration headaches and may involve other symptoms of external pathogens like runny nose, sneezing, or sore throat.

Internal: More gradual and chronic than external-type headaches, these headaches can be caused by either deficiency or excess in the meridians and organs. These are differentiated by the location and type of pain:

Locations:

Nape of neck/occiput: Kidney deficiency manifesting in the Urinary Bladder
Forehead: Stomach meridian excess or deficiency
Temples: Liver/Gallbladder excess
Top of head/vertex: Liver excess
Whole head: Qi deficiency

Types of pain:

Dull: Deficiency
Stabbing/throbbing: Stagnation
Heavy: Dampness/Phlegm

Treatments for headaches vary based on all of these potential manifestations. Acupuncture points on the head are almost always used to help disperse Qi, and your acupuncturist will use other distal points on the body to help keep Qi circulating. Tight muscles in the neck and shoulders can sometimes contribute to headaches, so your acupuncturist might use cupping or gua sha on your upper back to address that. In general, the more chronic the headaches, the longer it might take to see complete remission of headaches, but we like to see improvement in frequency and severity after a few visits.

Hot Flashes

Hot flashes are defined as the brief subjective or objective sensation of heat and are commonly experienced by women during menopause and just after childbirth. Hot flashes often occur in the evening or night and are accompanied by blushing and sweating; they can be very uncomfortable (and sometimes embarrassing). In Chinese medicine, hot flashes during menopause are almost always caused by a deficiency of Kidney Yin. Kidney Yin, which acts as a cooling factor in the body, declines as a woman reaches menopause, and this imbalance causes Yang to flare. We call this false Heat because it is caused by a deficiency of Yin, not an excess of Yang (Heat). Because Blood is a Yin substance, a Blood deficiency after giving birth can also lead to similar false Heat. Excess Heat in the Liver can also cause hot flashes, but these are usually accompanied by other signs of true Heat like red eyes and face, heavy sweating, and intense anger.

DIY Acupressure: Hot Flashes

The following points are useful for helping prevent and treat hot flashes. Using your fingertips, apply moderate pressure to each point for 60 to 90 seconds in a circular motion while taking deep, restorative breaths. Do this when you are experiencing a hot flash or twice daily for prevention.

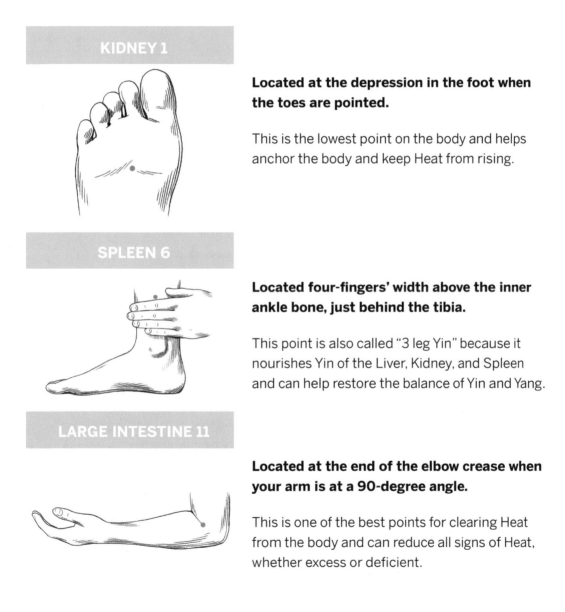

KIDNEY 1

Located at the depression in the foot when the toes are pointed.

This is the lowest point on the body and helps anchor the body and keep Heat from rising.

SPLEEN 6

Located four-fingers' width above the inner ankle bone, just behind the tibia.

This point is also called "3 leg Yin" because it nourishes Yin of the Liver, Kidney, and Spleen and can help restore the balance of Yin and Yang.

LARGE INTESTINE 11

Located at the end of the elbow crease when your arm is at a 90-degree angle.

This is one of the best points for clearing Heat from the body and can reduce all signs of Heat, whether excess or deficient.

Diagnosis and Treatment

The primary patterns we look for when treating issues with hot flashes are:

Kidney Yin Deficiency: Most common in perimenopause and menopause; hot flashes typically happen in the evening or at night, with or without sweating; typically accompanies dry skin and hair

Liver Heat: Hot flashes due to excess Heat; usually accompanies red face, red eyes, headache, temper

Blood Deficiency: More common in the postpartum months after childbirth and typically accompanies other symptoms like pallor, dizziness, dry skin and hair loss, and amenorrhea (absence of menstruation)

The patterns we look for when treating hot flashes can really differ, so it's important for an acupuncturist to look for other signs and symptoms that may be related, but a major clue can lie in the life stage of the patient. Postpartum and younger women tend to experience hot flashes due to Blood deficiency, menopausal women experience them due to Yin deficiency, and men typically experience them due to Liver Heat. Treatment plans typically include weekly visits until hot flashes become less frequent and less severe. Regular acupuncture during the transition into menopause is very helpful for many women to prevent hot flashes from occurring.

Insomnia

Insomnia is a sleep disorder characterized by an inability to fall asleep, stay asleep, or both. Insomnia can be very frustrating and can negatively impact daytime functioning, concentration, energy, and mood. Studies have shown that acupuncture can reduce anxiety, increase the production of melatonin (a hormone that regulates sleep-wake cycles), decrease the time it takes to fall asleep, and decrease nighttime waking—all this without the side effects, such as grogginess and dizziness, that conventional sleep-aid medications can cause.

In Traditional Chinese Medicine, quality and quantity of sleep directly relate to the Shen, so insomnia is categorized as a Shen disturbance. Because sleep is so important to all body functions (it's during sleep when Qi and Blood regenerate in the body), most acupuncturists will ask you about your sleep quantity and quality, regardless of whether or not it's the reason you're seeking treatment.

The Shen relies on Blood and Yin in the body, and thus on the Heart and the Liver, which store these substances. Because Yin is predominant at night, a deficiency of Yin will keep your body from resting. Blood is what houses the Shen, so a deficiency in Blood causes the Shen to "float," keeping it too active to adequately anchor. In my practice, Qi stagnation is the most common cause of insomnia, caused by overwork and our society's stressful demands.

Diagnosis and Treatment

The primary patterns we look for when treating insomnia are:

Liver Qi Stagnation: Difficulty staying asleep, waking between 1 and 3 a.m. (this is the Liver time on the Chinese medicine "organ clock"), vivid dreams, anxiety, irritability

Heart Blood Deficiency: Difficulty falling asleep, depression, anxiety, dizziness

Full-Heat Predominant: Restless sleep, frequent waking, subjective feeling of heat and excessive sweating; will also have signs of Heat during the day

Yin Deficiency: Waking several times throughout the night, night sweats, palpitations; common pattern during menopause

Improvements in sleep quality and quantity are some of the first signs that indicate the body is coming back into balance, so it's not unusual for a patient to notice improvements in sleep during the night following their acupuncture treatment. How long the improvement lasts depends on the severity of the issue. Chronic insomnia can take up to 8 to 10 treatments before seeing improvement, but during this course, other symptoms that are part of the presenting pattern of imbalance typically improve. An acute bout of insomnia might be nipped in just one session.

Your acupuncturist will probably suggest other ways to improve sleep, including turning off your cell phone and avoiding stimulating blue light from electronics for an hour before bedtime. If your mind races at night, your acupuncturist might recommend meditation or a foot soak before bed to help your Qi settle or gentle exercise like yoga to help your body and mind relax.

DIY Acupressure: Insomnia

The following acupressure points can be very helpful in supporting a good night's sleep. Using your fingertips, apply moderate pressure to each point for 60 to 90 seconds in a circular motion while taking deep, restorative breaths. It's best to use these points in the hour before bedtime.

KIDNEY 1

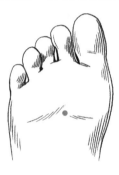

Located at the depression in the foot when the toes are pointed.

Because it is the lowest point on the body, this point is very grounding, especially for racing thoughts.

Tip: Applying lavender essential oil to this point right before bed can be very helpful for insomnia.

YIN TANG

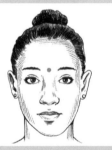

Located above the bridge of the nose between the eyebrows.

This point helps calm the Shen and relax the nervous system.

HEART 7

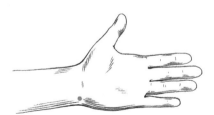

Located at the wrist crease, just inside the tendon that travels to the pinky finger.

This point nourishes the Heart, which in turn helps settle the Shen.

Jaw Problems

Jaw pain, clicking, clenching, and grinding (called temporomandibular dysfunction; TMD) can be very frustrating and uncomfortable. It can lead to other issue like headaches and difficulty chewing. Dental guards help protect your teeth from damage but do little to treat the cause of the issue. These issues can often be tied to Qi stagnation in the meridians that travel through the jaw, resulting in muscle tightness. Local and distal acupuncture is very effective in treating jaw problems.

Diagnosis and Treatment

The primary patterns we look for when treating jaw problems are:

Stomach Qi Stagnation: Local pain on lower jawline

Gallbladder Qi Stagnation: Jaw and temple pain

Liver Qi Stagnation: Jaw pain worse with stress and anxiety

Treatment for jaw problems will usually include local needling in the tight or painful area. This allows the muscle to release, and patients often feel instant relaxation and reduction in pain. The goal then is trying to get ahead of this pain and allow Qi to flow smoothly through the area.

Knee Pain

Knee pain is yet another common ailment that we tend to experience with age. In Chinese medicine, we believe this is because of the knee's involvement with the Kidney meridian. As our Kidney Essence and Qi decline with age, the Qi in the meridians can easily stagnate, causing pain. This pain is typically associated with chronic low back pain and may often accompany graying hair, dental issues, and bone fragility. Chronic knee pain that is worse with cold and damp weather can be due to Wind-Damp-Cold pathogens affecting the joints. Pain that is worse with heat and humidity is often due to Wind-Damp-Heat. Acute knee pain due to trauma or overuse is related to Qi and Blood stagnation.

Diagnosis and Treatment

The primary patterns we look for when treating knee pain are:

Qi Stagnation: Pain that seems to travel or switch knees, usually better with movement, often due to overuse (common in athletes and runners)

Blood Stagnation: Acute pain due to trauma (that is, tears to the ACL, MCL, or meniscus)

Kidney Qi Deficiency: Chronic, dull knee ache, often accompanied by backache

Wind-Damp-Cold: Stiff, achy pain worse with damp weather and alleviated by heat

Wind-Damp-Heat: Stiff, achy swollen knees worse with hot and humid weather and alleviated by cold

Depending on your diagnosis, your acupuncturist will choose points that treat the underlying pattern while also using local points on and around the knees to encourage Qi and Blood circulation. We always hope to see a reduction in pain in the first visit, but if pain is chronic, it may take several sessions to see results.

Memory and Concentration

Raise your hand if you've ever forgotten where you left your keys or searched far and wide for the sunglasses atop your head. If you suffer from brain fog, memory issues, inability to focus, or forgetfulness, you are not alone! A combination of poor diet, high stress, and not enough sleep can leave many of us feeling cloudy headed. And while we don't exactly know why, research has shown that acupuncture has a direct ability to influence brain activity, and recent studies suggest that acupuncture can be helpful in treating pre-dementia mild cognitive impairment.

In Chinese medicine, the brain is controlled by the Kidneys and is nourished by the Essence and Blood. The Kidneys control short-term memory and the ability to concentrate, so memory and concentration issues often have a relationship to an underlying Kidney deficiency. The Spleen also impacts memory and the ability to analyze and question. Patients who describe a feeling of heaviness and fogginess in the head often have issues with Dampness, which also point to a Spleen imbalance.

The Shen governs consciousness and emotions, and an imbalance here can cause insomnia, anxiety, and forgetfulness. Your acupuncturist will want to know specifics about your memory and concentration issues, such as when you tend to experience them, your quality and quantity of sleep, your stress level, and your digestion, which all can affect brain function.

Diagnosis and Treatment

The primary patterns we look for when treating memory and concentration issues are:

Kidney Qi and Essence Deficiency: Slowly declining memory, usually associated with age

Spleen Qi Deficiency with Dampness: "Brain fog" and heaviness; often worse after eating heavy or greasy meals

Blood Deficiency: Dizziness, insomnia; often seen in postpartum moms as "mommy brain"

Shen Disturbance: Concentration issues accompanied by anxiety, depression, and insomnia or other mental-health concerns

As mentioned earlier, acupuncture has a direct effect on the brain, and many people notice an improvement in their ability to concentrate in the days following acupuncture. (It's not uncommon to see students in acupuncture school studying for major exams with needles at the highest point on the top of the head.) For chronic issues with memory and concentration, several weekly treatments may be needed before seeing results.

Here's an acupressure tip: The point at the top of the head, called Du 20, is great for increasing concentration. It is found at the intersection of an imaginary line drawn from the tip of your nose and one drawn from the highest point of your ear. Using your fingertips, apply moderate pressure to this point for 60 to 90 seconds in circular motions. (And then go ace your exam or find your keys!)

Nausea

Nausea, with or without vomiting, is typically thought of as counterflow Qi, or Qi moving in the wrong direction. This is commonly seen during pregnancy, but many people also experience this in moving cars or on boats as well as during illness. If you've ever worn a seasickness band on your wrist while on a boat, you've already experienced acupressure! The bands are designed to press on an acupuncture point called

Pericardium 6 that calms nausea by correcting the flow of Qi in the torso. Counterflow Qi can be due to a temporary interruption in proper flow, due to the external physical bumpiness of a boat or car, or due to internal deficiencies or stagnations.

Nausea during pregnancy is usually due to the many changes in the body that occur during the first trimester that can temporarily impair proper Qi flow in the body. Morning sickness (or unfortunately, all-day sickness that many soon-to-be-mamas experience) can have aspects of Qi deficiency, Cold, Heat, or Dampness, and your acupuncturist will probably inquire about specific symptoms and the times of day you experience them to help identify the underlying patterns.

Chemotherapy-induced nausea is usually due to impairment of the Spleen and Stomach functions caused by medications. Nausea and vomiting can also result from overeating, eating too fast, and excess alcohol intake. These can cause Food stagnation and/or Stomach Heat, which pushes the Qi up in the wrong direction. Regardless of the cause, we can all agree that nausea is *no* fun. The good news is that acupuncture can effectively reduce nausea and vomiting by restoring proper Qi flow in the body.

Diagnosis and Treatment

The primary patterns we look for when treating nausea are:

Counterflow Qi: Nausea and vomiting, belching as seen in car and boat sickness and pregnancy; may be temporary or long lasting

Stomach and Spleen Qi Deficiency: Nausea, no appetite, feeling of heaviness in the body; common with chemotherapy-induced nausea and digestive disorders

Stomach Heat: Nausea, with a bitter or sour taste in the mouth, often due to medications, parasites, or excessive intake of alcohol

Food Stagnation: Common after a large, heavy meal, or after eating too fast; can also be due to excessive worry affecting the Spleen and Stomach

For treatment of nausea during pregnancy, weekly acupuncture is recommended until symptoms subside. Patients undergoing chemotherapy typically receive acupuncture during and after chemotherapy infusions, as those tend to be times when nausea is worse. For temporary symptoms, rest is usually the most helpful thing, and if you know you are prone to car or boat sickness, wearing those seasickness bands can help prevent nausea and vomiting.

Neck Tension and Pain

There's not much worse than waking up with a stiff neck or experiencing acute neck pain, hence the phrase "pain in the neck." Neck tension can easily lead to headaches and impaired range of motion and can make daily life challenging. Acupuncture can release tight muscles and allow for the smooth flow of Qi and Blood through the tissues. The backs of our necks are very susceptible to invasion by the external pathogen Wind, which can cause pain and stiffness, so many acupuncturists recommend wearing scarves on windy days to protect your neck and prevent stiffness.

Diagnosis and Treatment

The primary patterns we look for when treating neck pain are:

Qi Stagnation: Dull, achy pain that may travel through the neck or come and go through the day; might be due to spinal misalignment

Blood Stagnation: Pain in a fixed area, painful to the touch, usually due to trauma like whiplash

Wind Invasion: Stiff neck due to exposure to the external pathogen Wind

Structural issues and misalignment can be a major cause of neck pain, but muscle tightness can be either the cause or the compounding factor here, so acupuncture along with chiropractic manipulations tend to work best for neck pain. The more chronic the issue, the more treatments you may need. In addition to telling you to wear scarves, your acupuncturist will probably recommend that your neck is not exposed to Wind while you sleep—this means not sleeping too close to a fan, air conditioner, or open window.

Pregnancy

Nausea, heartburn, insomnia, constipation, and lower back pain are just some of the common issues that women experience during pregnancy. Luckily, acupuncture can help without the potentially harmful side effects caused by medications. Acupuncture is also commonly used to help turn breech babies, to get labor started, and to balance hormones in the postpartum period. Not all acupuncturists work with pregnant patients, and diagnosis can be a little bit different during this time, so make sure to work with someone who has experience treating pregnant women, and make sure their office setup can accommodate you comfortably, as it is advised that pregnant women don't lie flat on their backs during the later months of gestation.

Diagnosis and Treatment

These are some of the common patterns we see during pregnancy:

Counterflow Qi: Nausea, vomiting, heartburn

Liver Qi Stagnation: Pain, constipation, anxiety

Spleen Qi Deficiency: Fatigue, heavy legs, insomnia

The points your acupuncturist chooses will depend on what your symptoms and underlying pattern of disharmony are. Pregnancy itself is not an ailment, but the body goes through rapid changes and can function differently at this time, causing discomfort. In my practice, I like to see pregnant patients more regularly in the first trimester to promote a strong, healthy pregnancy and to prevent symptoms like nausea and fatigue, and at the end of the third trimester to help the body prepare for labor. In between those times, I recommend monthly preventive treatments or a short series of more regular visits to address any issues that arise.

There are a series of points used to help stimulate labor that are classically considered "forbidden" to use during pregnancy until the final weeks of the third trimester, so your acupuncturist will avoid these until you are full term. Don't be scared to try acupuncture while pregnant; it has a long, tried-and-tested safety record, but as with anything "new" during this time, always discuss your plans with your ob-gyn.

Stomachaches, Indigestion, and Heartburn

An occasional upset stomach or bout of indigestion is not uncommon and is usually caused by excessive food intake or stress. When this happens, a little hot water with ginger usually does the trick. Chronic gastrointestinal disorders like constipation, diarrhea, heartburn, IBS, and IBD all point to deeper imbalances in all of the organs and meridians that play a role in digestion, specifically the Stomach, Spleen, and Large Intestine. Acupuncture has been used for centuries to treat gastrointestinal issues, and research now shows that acupuncture might regulate gastrointestinal motility (the movement of the digestive system) and reduce pain by helping balance the two branches of the autonomic nervous system by stimulating the vagus nerve, one of the most important nerves in the body.

Diagnosis and Treatment

The primary patterns we look for when treating digestive issues are:

Spleen Qi Deficiency: Bloating, indigestion, fatigue, diarrhea, low appetite, vague feeling of fullness

Stomach Heat: Intense hunger, thirst, belching, nausea, heartburn

Liver Qi Stagnation Affecting the Spleen: Diarrhea or constipation worse with stress, upper abdominal pain, and distention

Yin and Body Fluids Deficiency: Constipation with dry, hard stools

Damp-Heat in the Stomach and Large Intestine: Urgent, foul-smelling stools accompanied by sensation of heat; might see mucus in stools; discomfort alleviated by bowel movements

In addition to acupuncture treatments, your acupuncturist may prescribe herbs that are known to regulate the digestive processes and may also recommend dietary changes. In Chinese medicine, the intake of energetically Cold foods can damage the digestive tract, so your acupuncturist might recommend cooking or steaming vegetables and limiting your intake of icy, cold beverages. Adding warming spices like ginger and cinnamon to the diet can also be helpful for digestive issues. Excessively hot, spicy, and fried foods, as well as alcohol, can contribute to Stomach Heat and lead to heartburn, so if this is your main issue, your acupuncturist may advise you to avoid these foods.

Weight Loss

While there is no "magic" acupuncture point for weight loss (believe me, lots of people ask!), acupuncture can help get to the root of imbalances that might be preventing you from losing weight. Your acupuncturist will ask several questions about other areas of your health to create a picture of your overall wellness. Stress hormones tell the body to hold on to fat, so working to reduce stress can often have a big impact.

The other area we often look at is digestion. If your digestion is slow, you may not be metabolizing food properly, which can make it difficult to lose weight. In Chinese medicine, this is a hallmark Spleen Qi deficiency. Hormonal balance (regulated by the Kidneys) is also important in weight regulation, so it's another area we will examine.

Cravings for certain foods can often signify imbalances in specific organs: Sugar cravings relate to the Spleen, salt cravings relate to the Kidney, and sour cravings relate to the Liver. There are also several points on the ear that are known for their effectiveness in resolving cravings.

Diagnosis and Treatment

The primary patterns we look for when hoping to promote weight loss are:

Spleen Qi Deficiency with Dampness: Sugar cravings, abdominal bloating, low muscle tone, fatigue

Kidney Yang Deficiency: Edema, low back pain, hormonal imbalance, frequent urination, sensation of cold, salt cravings

Liver Qi Stagnation: Irritability, cold hands and feet, sour cravings, high stress

If you are seeking treatment to help you lose weight, your acupuncturist will evaluate all the other systems of your body and look for signs of imbalance. The goal is to make sure you are digesting and eliminating properly, sleeping enough, have balanced hormones, and aren't experiencing too much stress. Working to improve these areas often results in weight loss.

Acupuncture for weight loss typically involves two or more treatments a week for the first few weeks and then tapering down when you begin to meet your goals. Ear acupuncture is often used to reduce cravings. Of course, committing to a clean diet and regular exercise is an important factor here, so I also like to refer patients coming to me for weight loss to trainers, nutritionists, and health coaches for best results.

Wrist Pain

Thanks in part to the introduction of handheld technology into our everyday lives, wrist pain is on the rise. Frequent texting, emailing, game playing, and "liking" on our smartphones is causing damage to our thumb tendons, which connect the thumb to the forearm. (And you thought the only possible risk of all that "swiping left" on dating apps was heartache!) Spending too much time typing on a keyboard or clicking a mouse can often cause burning, tingling pain in the wrist and hand called carpal tunnel syndrome. Wrist pain can also be caused by arthritis, injuries, and other inflammatory conditions. Wrist pain and carpal tunnel syndrome are becoming common ailments that drive people to seek out acupuncture.

Acupuncture can help restore proper Qi and Blood flow to the wrist and can reduce pain and inflammation. In fact, a 2011 study found acupuncture to be more effective at treating carpal tunnel pain than steroid injections.

Diagnosis and Treatment

The primary patterns we look for when treating wrist pain are:

Qi Stagnation: Achy pain that travels and might switch sides

Blood Stagnation: Pain due to trauma, injury, or overuse

Blood Deficiency: Tingling and numbness

Wind-Damp-Cold: Pain worse with cold and damp days, sensation of heaviness, alleviated by heat

Wind-Damp-Heat: Pain worse with hot and humid days, sensation of heaviness, alleviated by cold

Treatment for wrist pain usually involves local needles to help disperse stagnant Qi and Blood and to reduce inflammation and decrease pain, as well as other points on the body to encourage proper flow of Qi. If your wrist pain is caused by computer or phone use, your acupuncturist will probably suggest limiting the time you use these devices or taking breaks throughout the day. For chronic issues, it may take several acupuncture treatments before seeing results, but with acute pain and trauma, you may start seeing results after just one visit.

Glossary

Acupuncture: The primary therapeutic method of Chinese medicine in which insertion of a hair-thin needle into a specific point on the body is used to promote balance and healing via activation and regulation of Qi.

Cun: Body inch; the proportional measurement used to locate acupuncture points on the body.

Cupping: A Chinese medicine therapy in which glass or plastic cups are applied to the body with suction to relieve stagnation and promote flow of Qi and Blood through the tissues.

Essence: A vital substance of the body that influences one's constitution, potential, development, and reproduction; also known as Jing.

External pathogen: A cause of disease that originates outside of the body; the six external pathogens in Chinese medicine are Wind, Cold, Heat, Dryness, Dampness, and Summer Heat.

Gua sha: A Chinese medicine technique in which the skin is scraped with a smooth tool to promote blood flow to the tissues.

Meridian: A pathway or channel in the body along which Qi flows.

Moxibustion: A Chinese medicine therapy in which dried mugwort is burned over an area of the body or needle to reduce pain and promote blood flow.

Needled/Needling: The act of receiving or performing acupuncture.

Organ clock: Qi circulates through the body in 24-hour cycles. Each of the 12 organs is dominant during a two-hour segment, and these segments make up the organ clock. If a patient has specific symptoms at the same time every day, the acupuncturist might take note of the associated organ on the organ clock.

Pattern: A grouping of related symptoms that is used to form a diagnosis.

Point prescription: The set of points used in an acupuncture treatment.

Qi: "Vital energy" or "life force" that circulates through the body in the meridians and is manipulated by acupuncture.

Shen: The spirit, consciousness, and emotional component of the body.

Wei Qi: The protective Qi in the body, most closely related to immunity.

Yang: The hot, active, hollow, and bright aspects of the body and environment.

Yin: The cool, slow, solid, and dark aspects of the body and environment.

Resources

ACAOM (Accreditation Commission for Acupuncture and Oriental Medicine Directory of Accredited Programs)

acaom.org/directory-menu/directory/

This is a list of all accredited acupuncture programs.

Acupuncture Now Foundation

www.acunow.org

The ANF is a leader in the collection and dissemination of unbiased and authoritative information about all aspects of the practice of acupuncture.

NCCAOM Find a Practitioner Directory

www.nccaom.org/find-a-practitioner-directory/

This is a database of all board-certified acupuncturists in the United States.

Pacific College of Oriental Medicine

pacificcollege.edu

This is my alma mater and one of the largest acupuncture programs in the United States, with campuses in New York City, Chicago, and San Diego.

FURTHER READING

Between Heaven and Earth: A Guide to Chinese Medicine, by Harriet Beinfield and Efrem Korngold

The Spark in the Machine, by Daniel Keown

The Web That Has No Weaver, by Ted Kaptchuk

References

Abenyakar, Sefkat, and Feyza Boneval. "Increased Plasma β-Endorphin Concentrations after Acupuncture: Comparison of Electroacupuncture, Traditional Chinese Acupuncture, Tens and Placebo Tens." *Acupuncture in Medicine* 12, no. 1 (May 1994): 21–23. doi: 10.1136/aim.12.1.21.

Al-Bedah, Abdullah M. N., Ibrahim S. Elsubai, Naseem Akhtar Qureshi, Tamer Shaban Aboushanab, Gazzaffi I. M. Ali, Ahmed Tawfik El-Olemy, Asim A. H. Khalil, Mohamed K. M. Khalil, and Meshari Saleh Alqaed. "The Medical Perspective of Cupping Therapy: Effects and Mechanisms of Action." *Journal of Traditional and Complementary Medicine* 9, no. 2 (April 2019): 90–97. doi: 10.1016/j.jtcme.2018.03.003.

Amorim, Diogo, José Amado, Irma Brito, Sónia M. Fiuza, Nicole Amorim, Cristina Costeira, and Jorge Machado. "Acupuncture and Electroacupuncture for Anxiety Disorders: A Systematic Review of the Clinical Research." *Complementary Therapies in Clinical Practice* 31 (May 2018): 31–37. doi: 10.1016/j.ctcp.2018.01.008.

Bauer, Matthew, and Mel Hopper Koppelman. "Acupuncture: More than Pain Management." *White Paper*, Acupuncture Now Foundation. Accessed April 3, 2019. www.acunow.org/white-papers.html.

Bauke, Nicole. "Battlefield Acupuncture? Yes, It Exists, and the Military Is Using It to Fight Troops' Pain." *Military Times*. February 10, 2018. Accessed April 1, 2019. www.militarytimes.com/news/your-military/2018/02/09/battlefield-acupuncture-yes-it-exists-and-the-military-is-using-it-to-fight-troops-pain/.

Berman, Brian M., Lixing Lao, Patricia Langenberg, Wen Lin Lee, Adele M. K. Gilpin, and Marc C. Hochberg. "Effectiveness of Acupuncture as Adjunctive Therapy in Osteoarthritis of the Knee: A Randomized, Controlled Trial." *Annals of Internal Medicine* 141, no. 12 (December 2004): 901–10. doi: 10.7326/0003-4819-141-12-200412210-00006.

Cao, Huijuan, Xingfang Pan, Hua Li, and Jianping Liu. "Acupuncture for Treatment of Insomnia: A Systematic Review of Randomized

Controlled Trials." *The Journal of Alternative and Complementary Medicine* 15, no. 11 (November 2009): 1171–86. doi: 10.1089/acm.2009.0041.

Chan, Yuan-Yu, Wan-Yu Lo, Szu-Nian Yang, Yi-Hung Chen, and Jaung-Geng Lin. "The Benefit of Combined Acupuncture and Antidepressant Medication for Depression: A Systematic Review and Meta-Analysis." *Journal of Affective Disorders* 176 (May 2015): 106–17. doi: 10.1016/j.jad.2015.01.048.

Chen, Longyun, Anli Xu, Nina Yin, Min Zhao, Zhigang Wang, Tao Chen, Yisheng Gao, and Zebin Chen. "Enhancement of Immune Cytokines and Splenic CD4+ T Cells by Electroacupuncture at ST36 Acupoint of SD Rats." *PLoS One* 12, no. 4 (April 2017): e0175568. doi: 10.1371/journal.pone.0175568.

Deng, Min, and Xu-Feng Wang. "Acupuncture for Amnestic Mild Cognitive Impairment: A Meta-Analysis of Randomised Controlled Trials." *Acupuncture in Medicine* 34, no. 5 (October 2016): 342–48. doi: 10.1136/acupmed-2015-010989.

Dhond, Rupali P., Calvin Yeh, Kyungmo Park, Norman Kettner, and Vitaly Napadow. "Acupuncture Modulates Resting State Connectivity in Default and Sensorimotor Brain Networks." *Pain* 136, no. 3 (June 2008): 407–18. doi: 10.1016/j.pain.2008.01.011.

Haake, Michael, Hans-Helge Müller, Carmen Schade-Brittinger, Heinz D. Basler, Helmut Schäfer, Christoph Maier, Heinz G. Endres, Hans J. Trampisch, and Albrecht Molsberger. "German Acupuncture Trials (Gerac) For Chronic Low Back Pain: Randomized, Multicenter, Blinded, Parallel-Group Trial With 3 Groups." *Archives of Internal Medicine* 167, no. 17 (2007): 1892–98. doi: 10.1001/Archinte.167.17.1892.

Han, Ji-Sheng. "Acupuncture and Endorphins." *Neuroscience Letters* 361, no. 1–3 (May 2004): 258–61. doi: 10.1016/j.neulet.2003.12.019.

Hui, Kathleen K. S., Jing Liu, Nikos Makris, Randy L. Gollub, Anthony J. W. Chen, Christopher I. Moore, David N. Kennedy, Bruce R. Rosen, and Kenneth K. Kwong. "Acupuncture Modulates the Limbic System and Subcortical Gray Structures of the Human Brain: Evidence from fMRI

Studies in Normal Subjects." *Human Brain Mapping* 9, no. 1 (2000): 13–25. doi: 10.1002/(SICI)1097-0193(2000)9:1<13::AID-HBM2>3.0.CO;2-F.

Ji-Sheng, Han. "Acupuncture and Endorphins." *Neuroscience Letters* 361, no 1–3 (May 2004): 258–61. doi: 10.1016/j.neulet.2003.12.019.

Keown, Daniel. *The Spark in the Machine: How the Science of Acupuncture Explains the Mysteries of Western Medicine.* London: Singing Dragon, 2014.

Koppelman, Mel Hopper. "Acupuncture: An Overview of Scientific Evidence." *Evidence Based Acupuncture.* Accessed May 06, 2019. https://www.evidencebasedacupuncture.org/present-research/acupuncture-scientific-evidence/.

Linde, Klaus, Gianni Allais, Benno Brinkhaus, Yutong Fei, Michael Mehring, Emily A. Vertosick, Andrew Vickers, and Adrian R. White. "Acupuncture for the Prevention of Episodic Migraine." *Cochrane Database of Systematic Reviews* 2016, no. 6 (June 2016). doi: 10.1002/14651858.CD001218.pub3.

Linde, Klaus, Gianni Allais, Benno Brinkhaus, Yutong Fei, Michael Mehring, Byung-Cheul Shin, Andrew Vickers, and Adrian R. White. "Acupuncture for the Prevention of Tension–Type Headache." *Cochrane Database of Systematic Reviews* 2016, no. 4 (April 2016). doi: 10.1002/14651858.CD007587.pub2.

McDonald, John, and Stephen Janz. *The Acupuncture Evidence Project: A Comparative Literature Review.* Revised ed. Brisbane, Australia: Australian Acupuncture and Chinese Medicine Association Ltd., 2017.

National Institutes of Health. "The National Institutes of Health Consensus Development Conference Statement: Acupuncture." November 3–5, 1997. Accessed April 3, 2019. consensus.nih.gov/1997/1997acupuncture107html.htm.

Paulus, Wolfgang E., Mingmin Zhang, Erwin Strehler, Imam El-Danasouri, and Karl Sterzik. "Influence of Acupuncture on the Pregnancy Rate in Patients Who Undergo Assisted Reproduction Therapy." *Fertility and Sterility* 77, no. 4 (April 1, 2002): 721–24. doi: 10.1016/S0015-0282(01)03273-3.

Siterman, S., F. Eltes, V. Wolfson, H. Lederman, and B. Bartoov. "Does Acupuncture Treatment Affect Sperm Density in Males with Very Low Sperm Count? A Pilot Study." *Andrologia* 32, no. 1 (January 2000): 31–39. doi: 10.1111/j.1439-0272.2000.tb02862.x.

Spence, D. Warren, Leonid Kayumov, Adam Chen, Alan Lowe, Umesh Jain, Martin A. Katzman, Jianhua Shen, Boris Perelman, and Colin M. Shapiro. "Acupuncture Increases Nocturnal Melatonin Secretion and Reduces Insomnia and Anxiety: A Preliminary Report." *The Journal of Neuropsychiatry and Clinical Neurosciences* 16, no. 1 (February 2004): 19–28. doi: 10.1176/jnp.16.1.19.

Takahashi, Toku. "Chapter Fourteen—Effect and Mechanism of Acupuncture on Gastrointestinal Diseases." *International Review of Neurobiology* 111 (2013): 273–94. doi: 10.1016/B978-0-12-411545-3.00014-6.

Wang, Xiaoyu, Hong Shi, Hongyan Shang, Wei He, Shuli Chen, Gerhard Litscher, Ingrid Gaischek, and Xianghong Jing. "Effect of Electroacupuncture at ST36 on Gastric-Related Neurons in Spinal Dorsal Horn and Nucleus Tractus Solitarius." *Evidence-Based Complementary and Alternative Medicine* 2013 (2013). doi: 10.1155/2013/912898.

Yang, Chun-Pai, Nai-Hwei Wang, Tsai-Chung Li, Ching-Liang Hsieh, Hen-Hong Chang, Kai-Lin Hwang, Wang-Sheng Ko, and Ming-Hong Chang. "A Randomized Clinical Trial of Acupuncture Versus Oral Steroids for Carpal Tunnel Syndrome: A Long-Term Follow-Up." *The Journal of Pain* 12, no. 2 (February 2011): 272–79. doi: 10.1016/j.jpain.2010.09.001.

Index

Acknowledgments

To all the teachers, past and present, who have dedicated their lives to sharing the gift of Chinese medicine and advocating for its acceptance: Thank you, I know it wasn't always easy.

To Callisto Media, and especially to my editor Rachel Feldman: Thank you for realizing the need for this book and for inviting me on this journey!

Randie: You are the foundation on which I have built my dreams. Thank you for your unwavering support and love.

Sadie and Remy: You are my sunshine. Thank you for filling me with joy and pride.

To my Brownies: I love you all to the sky and back.

To my incredible network of friends, old and new: Thank you for your support and encouragement.

To my colleagues, especially Caitlin Donovan, who opened the door to Chinese medicine for me, and Elissa Ranney, who helps my business wheels turn smoothly: Thank you!

To my patients at Indigo Acupuncture + Wellness: Thank you for letting me share in your lives and your stories and for trusting in me with your care. I am so grateful for you and honored to work with you.

About the Author

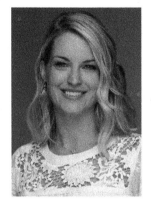

Sarah Swanberg, **MS LAc**, is a Licensed Acupuncturist and Board Certified Diplomate in Oriental Medicine through the NCCAOM. She holds a Master of Science in Traditional Oriental Medicine from the Pacific College of Oriental Medicine in New York City. In her practice, Indigo Acupuncture + Wellness, located in Stamford, Connecticut, Sarah combines the time-honored art of Chinese medicine with practical health advice for the modern world. She lives in Stamford, Connecticut, with her husband and two daughters. You can find her at indigoacu.com or on Instagram at @indigoacu.